SṚIṢTI

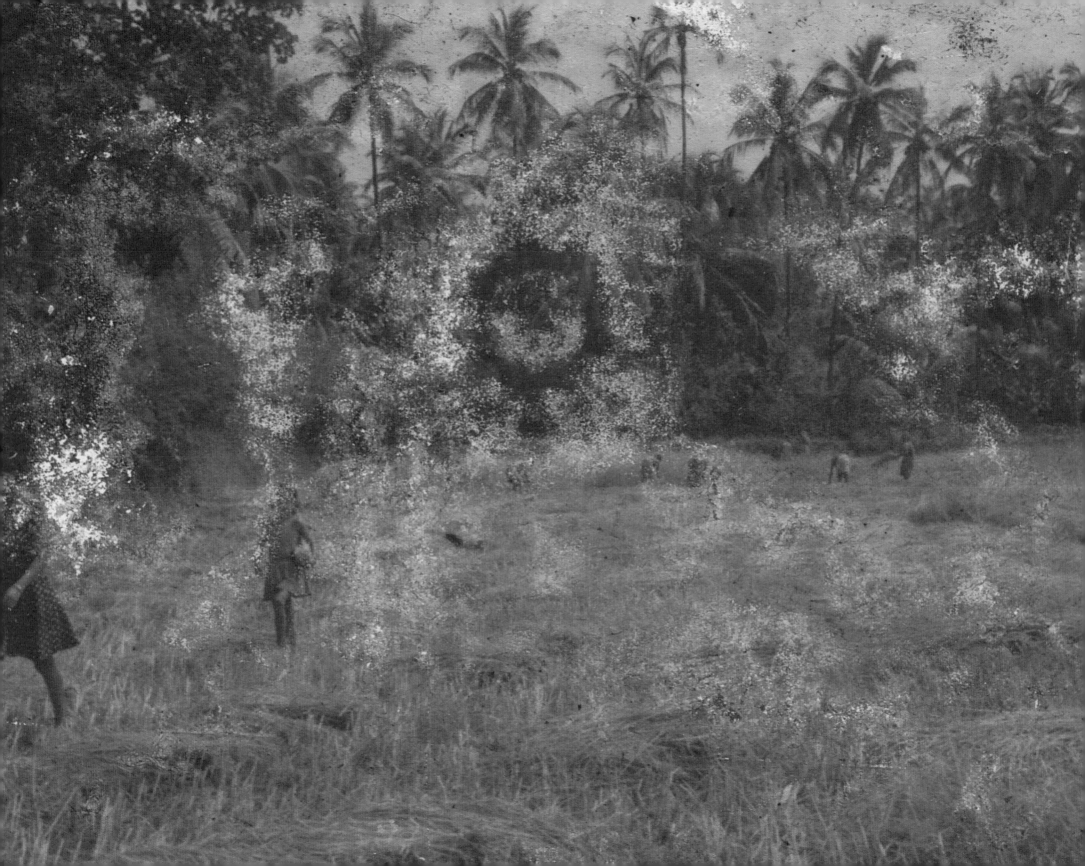

SṚIṢṬI

Sharmila Desai

Dance and Performance

foreword by
Trudie Styler and Sting

with essays by
**Karole Armitage
Olivier Berggruen
Jeffrey Deitch**

Edited by
Olivier Berggruen

TROLLEY

special thanks:
Guruji Sri K. Pattabhi Jois and Sharath Rangaswamy, Guru Frey,
Joseph Torczon, Desais, Sumners, Olivier Berggruen, Max Hollein,
Sharifa Rhodes-Pitts, Torczons, Rangaswamys, Jeffrey Deitch,
Karole Armitage, Shahzia Sikkander, Michael Weinfeld, VPL Victoria
Bartlett, Mo-Ling Chui, Pirashanna Thevaraja, Bangalore Prakash,
Mr Balachandar, Brooke Slezak, Vanina Sorrenti, Briana Blasko,
Paul Breen, Max Vadukul and Nicoletta Santoro, Ai-Jen Poo, Jee Kim,
Waleed Khairzada, Italo Zucchelli, Mary Frey, Tom Sachs, Hendrys,
Scotts & Richard Spahn

Published in Great Britain in 2006
by Trolley Ltd
73a Redchurch Street, London E2 7DJ, UK
www.trolleybooks.com

ISBN 1-904563-50-3

Designed by Sharmila Desai
in collaboration with Michael Ian Weinfeld

Editor: Olivier Berggruen; Assistant Editor: Sharifa Rhodes-Pitts

for
my family

foreword

When we met Sharmila, she came into our lives and quietly, organically, took her special place in the lives of the whole family. It is difficult to describe her in ordinary terms, because they would ground her and make her of the earth, and she is not quite of the earth.

Within her graceful and tiny form a great spirit is barely contained, giving her an ethereal and powerful energy. As the light changes, she changes. She is at once old and young. She is a fabulous and exotic creature who has accidentally found her way out of Paradise.

When she teaches you are in the company of an ancient. When she dances she transforms herself, the goddess emerges and the watcher is transfixed. A beautiful being on whom God shines his light. She is goodness, she is kindness, she is as noble as she is simple. She moves with grace, she embodies grace. There it is: Sharmila Desai is Grace.

We suggest you see and read this book and you will glimpse her extraordinary nature for yourself.

Trudie Styler and Sting

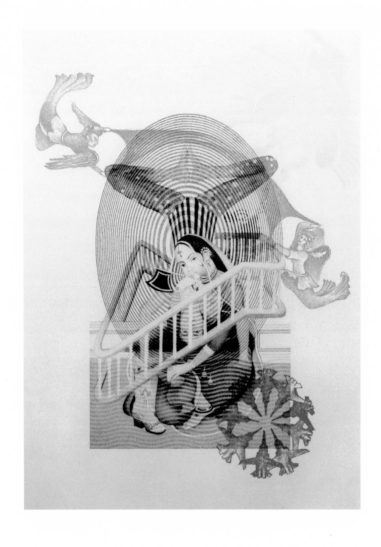

SṚIṢṬI

In Indian worship, yantra – a pure geometric
diagram – is a tool to stimulate inner visualizations,
meditations and experiences.

One of the predominant elementary diagrams is the
triangle, or trikona. The primary triangle represents
the three fold process of creation [sristi],
preservation [sthithi] and dissolution [samhara].

This book is an offering to the creative principle, SṚIṢṬI.

KAROLE ARMITAGE

The first time I saw Sharmila practicing yoga I was amazed. Her ability to control her body with awe-inspiring precision was mysterious. How could she stand on her hands for several minutes and command her legs to move in a long series of different positions without falling over? How could she achieve an extreme level of flexibility without a hint of force as her body folded into impossible positions? And most astonishing of all, how could she roll over and over again on the floor as if levitated, skimming the baseboards with only her head and feet touching the ground?

As a choreographer and dancer, I have spent my life studying the ways in which the human body can be used as a finely tuned instrument. I found Sharmila's choreography very familiar and very different from the way a ballet dancer creates form. I gradually realized that yoga, like ballet, is based on an understanding of the skeletal system in combination with the laws of physics. But there is one fundamental difference: dance is made for others, yoga is done for oneself. This difference is manifested in the way yoga uses isometric motion to create balance and strength whereas ballet uses positions and rhythm to move beyond the apparent limitations of the body.

In yoga, all movements are rooted in the human body's skeletal and muscular systems. Yoga works out of the body's architecture on a geometric level, which gives it a feeling of great purity. It is somehow deeply grounded in our universe. Though ballet is based on the same naturalness and purity, it requires a level of speed and technique that make it exciting and communicative to an audience. Ballet produces a different way of controlling the forces of gravity. The two techniques have a lot in common and yet are very different: yoga is about practice and ballet is about performance.

Sharmila Desai is bridging the gap between practice and performance. Her work, like Indian culture, is of a composite nature. The coming together of great civilizations of the Middle East and South Asia under Muslim rule produced new hybrids in all spheres of life in India. In music, the long-necked Persian lute was combined with the Indian vina to form the sitar. In architecture, the monumental buildings of the Mughals, such as the Taj Mahal, reconciled the indigenous Hindu style with the arch and dome of Islam, producing a fusion more beautiful than either predecessor. Sharmila similarly merges different aspects of Indian culture into a new form for the stage. She introduces elements of the Keralan martial arts known as *Kalaripayattu* and aspects of *Bharata-Natyam*, one of the classical dance forms of India, with her Ashtanga yoga practice.

Sharmila's quiet and powerful concentration makes her slowly evolving, rock-solid shapes appear like sculpture. The tempo is slow enough and the effect is grounded so deeply in nature, that she appears still even while in motion. The depth of her concentration makes her seem beyond personality, like an ancient figure carved in stone. The effect of her silence is profound, yet mystifying and communicative. By uniting the rich heritage of dance, martial arts, and yoga in an unforeseen way, Sharmila is guiding performance into new territory.

Om Bhur Bhuvan Svah
Tat Savithur varenyam
Bhargo Devasya Dheemahi
Dhiyo Yo Nah Prachodayat

GAYATRI MANTRA

The Rig Veda (10:16:3)

'From the unreal [asat]
lead me to the real [sat]!
From the darkness lead me to light!
From death lead me to immorality!'

Traditionally, Indian ritual art is a way of sharing sadhana, one's progressive unification
with the vital principle… It is an experience, daily repeated, which leads towards integration,
and to an expansion of consciousness which gives rise to perception of the whole…

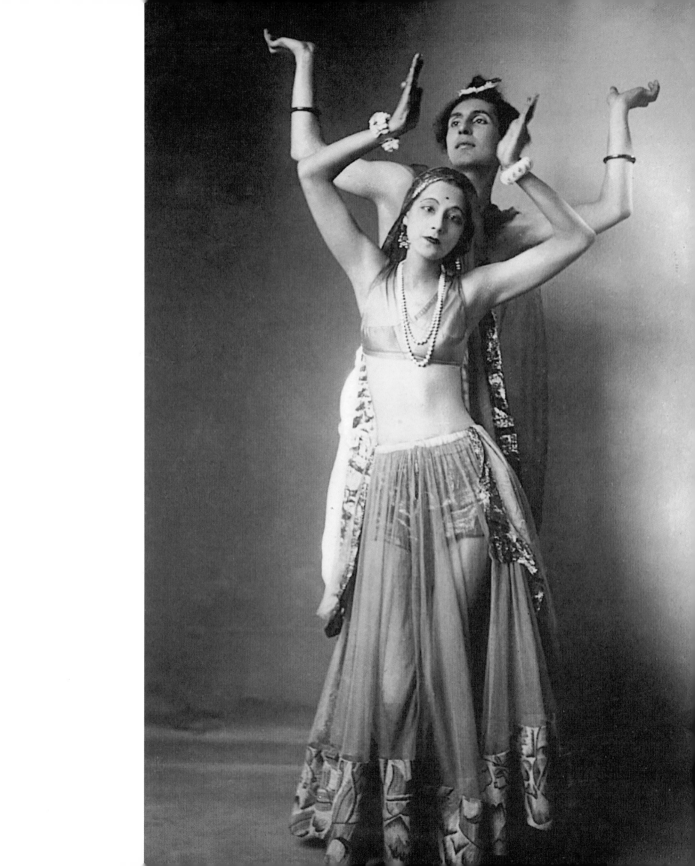

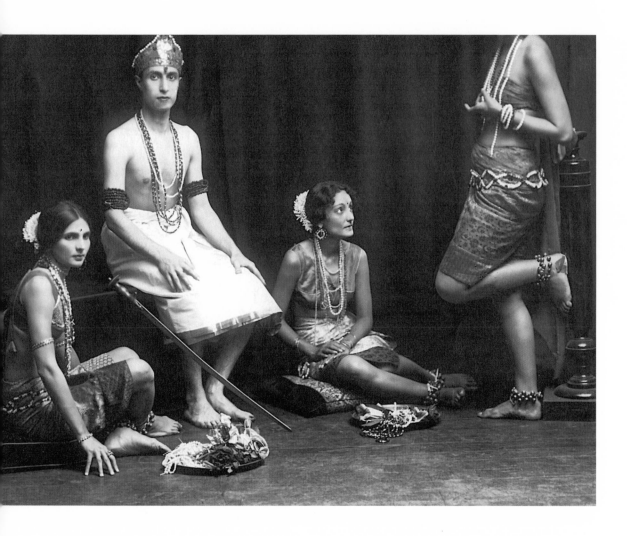

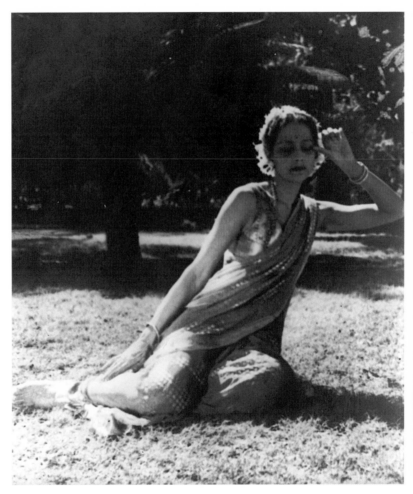
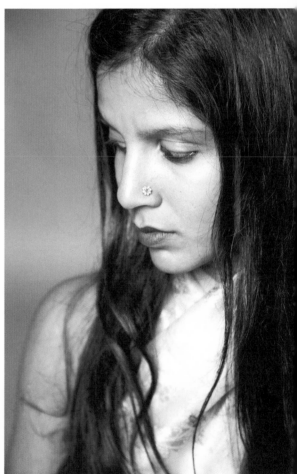

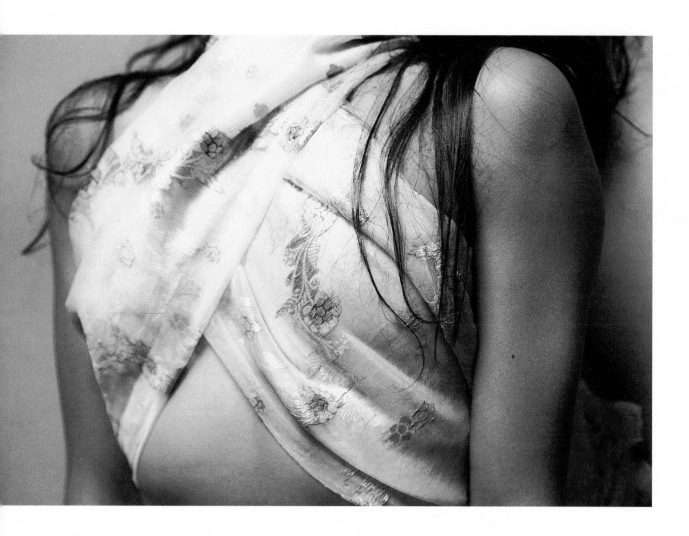

V

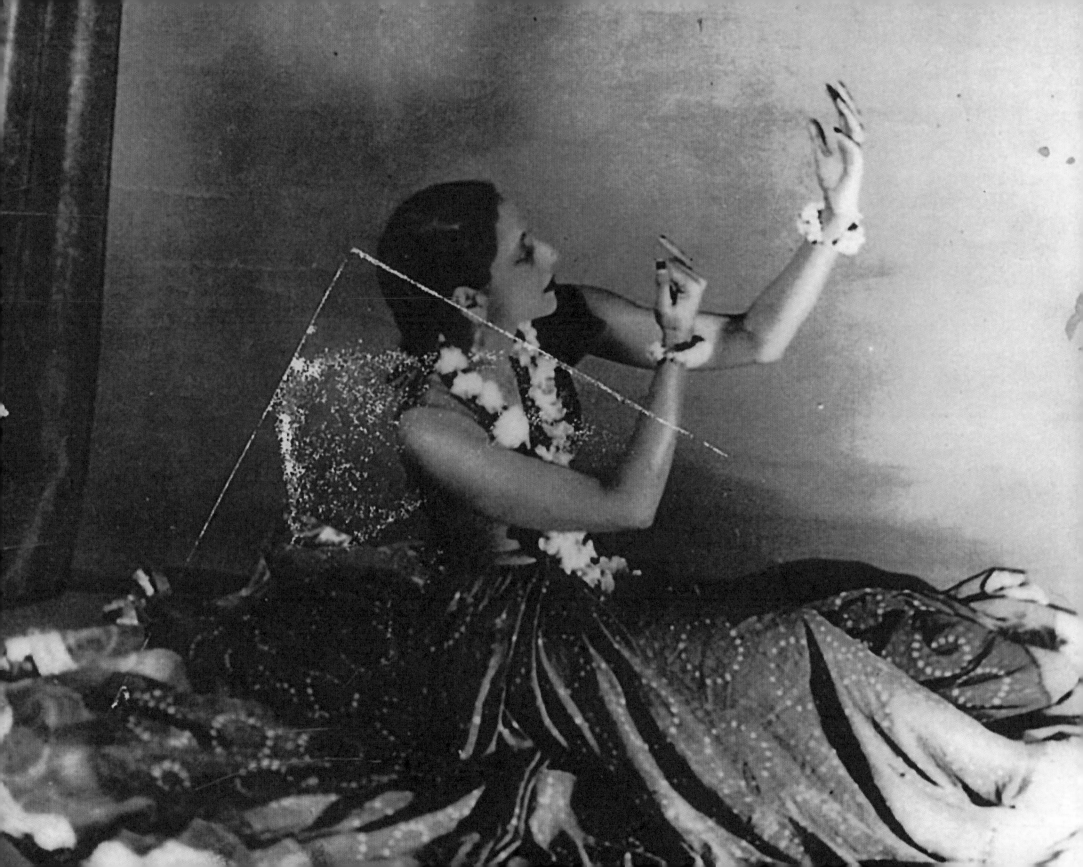

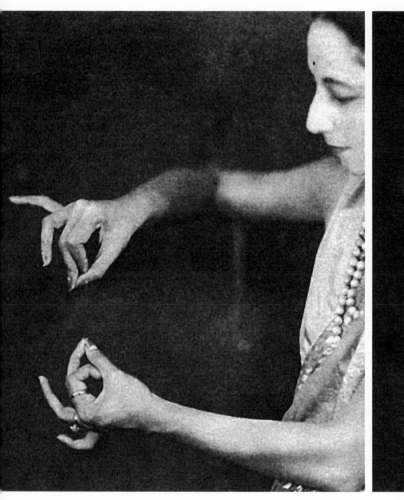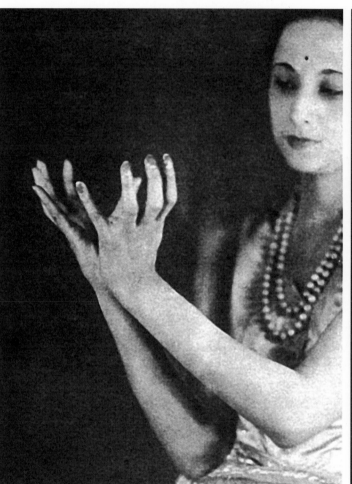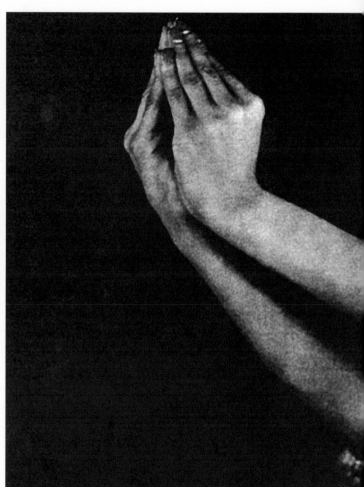

… To dissolve oneself systematically into the essence – this is the unifying purpose of all Indian ritual. The ritual impulse everywhere is essentially an impulse towards reverence of the life-force and self-identification with it…

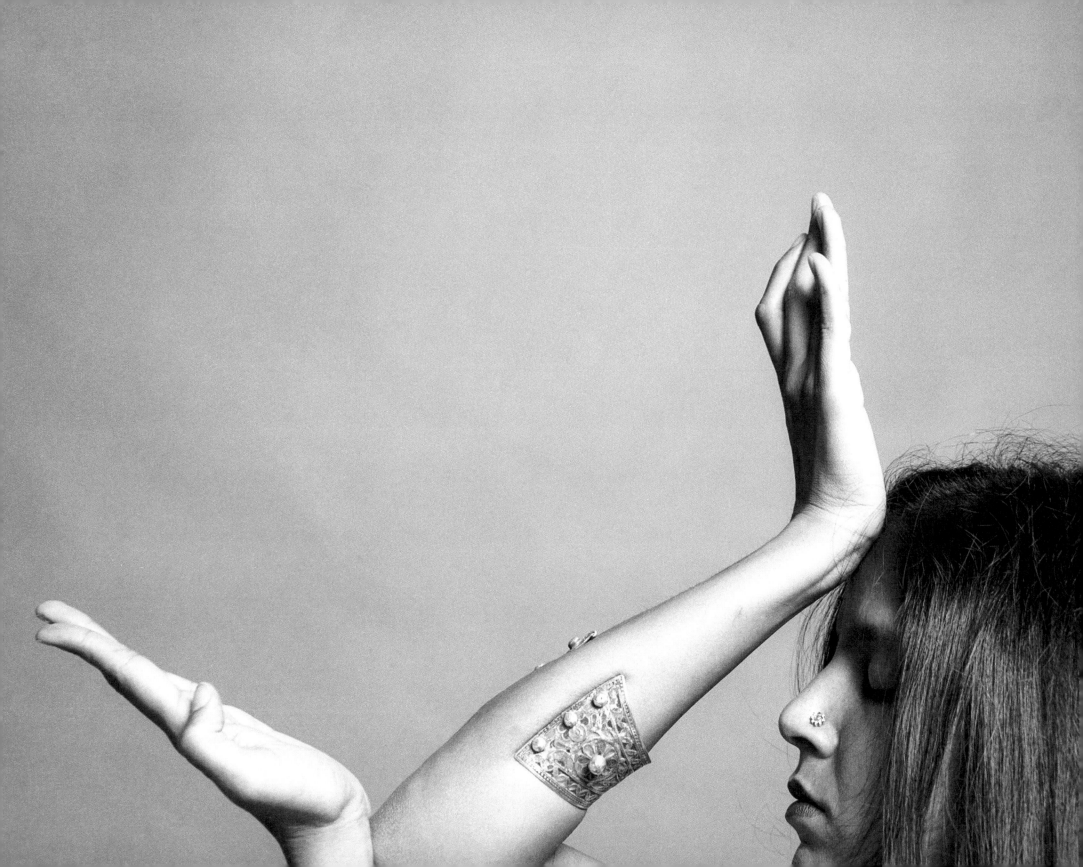

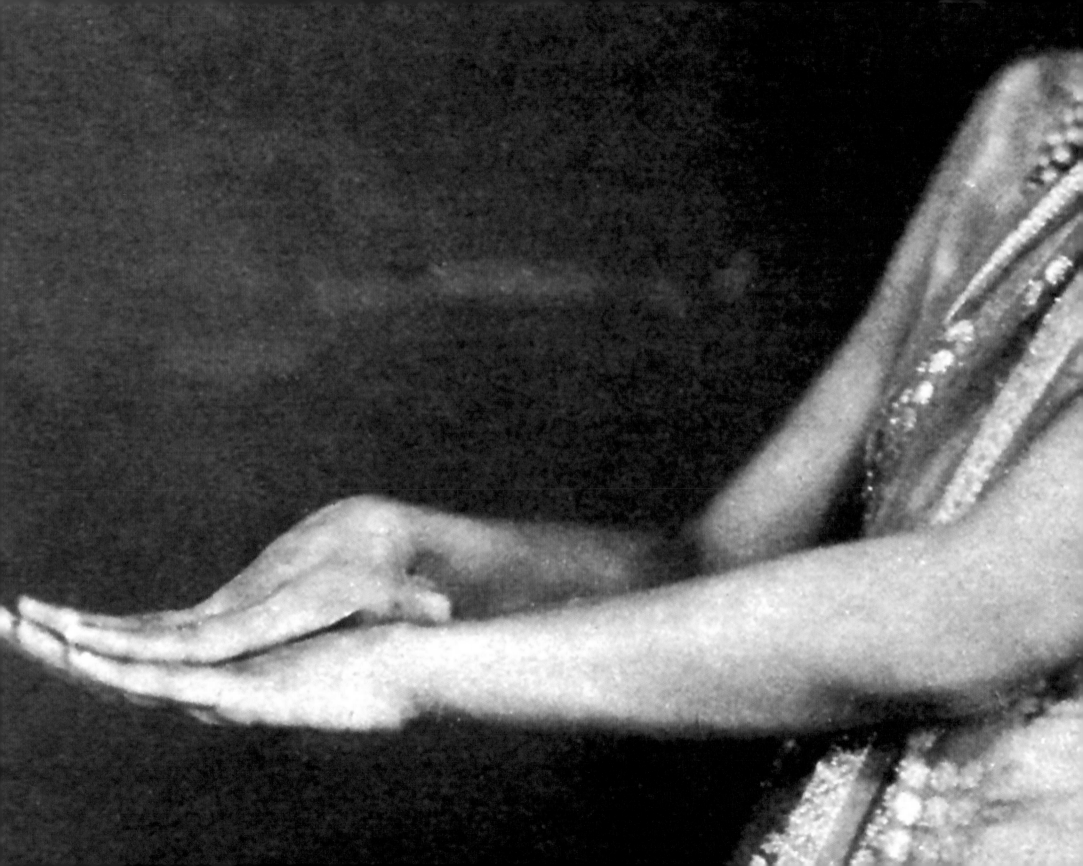

… Daily rites include the greeting of the sun at its rising – a cycle of yogic and ritual gestures directed towards the east and accompanied by prescribed mantras – the offering of grain and clarified butter to the pure flame, and the sandhya or twilight prayers, recited as dusk falls when lamps are lighted in every traditional home to the sound of bell and gong.

AJIT MOOKERJEE

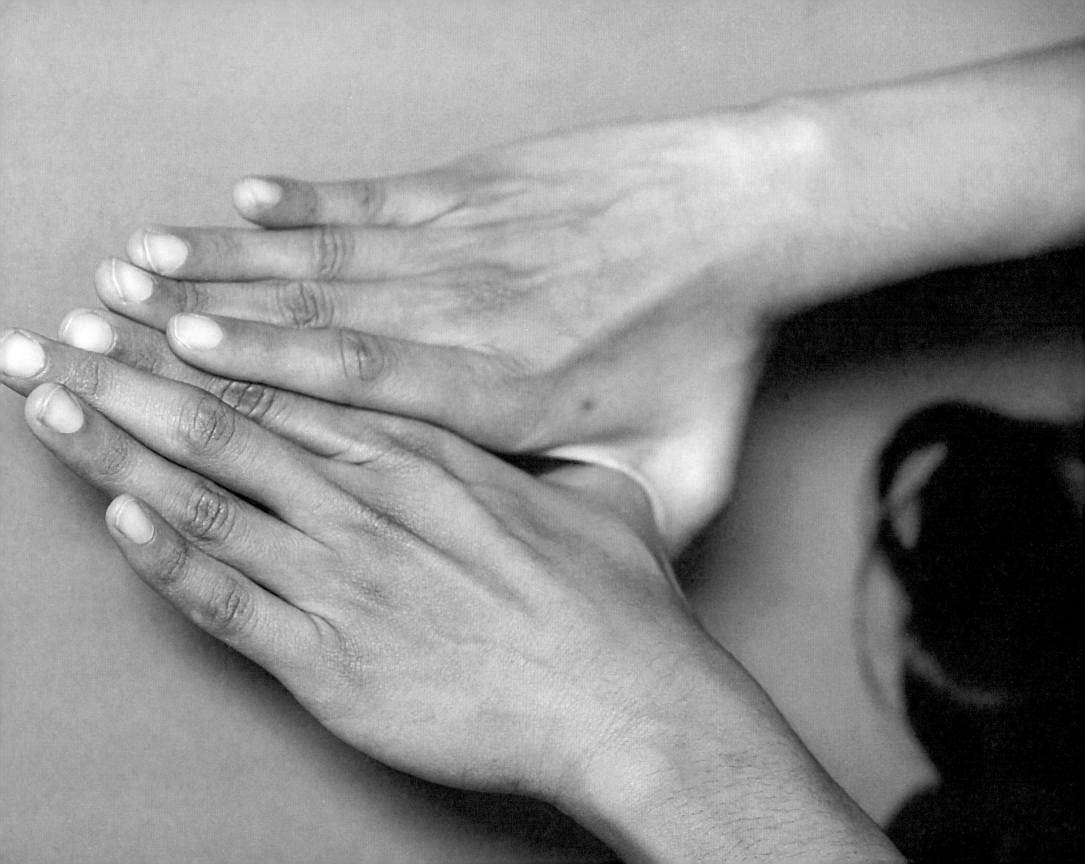

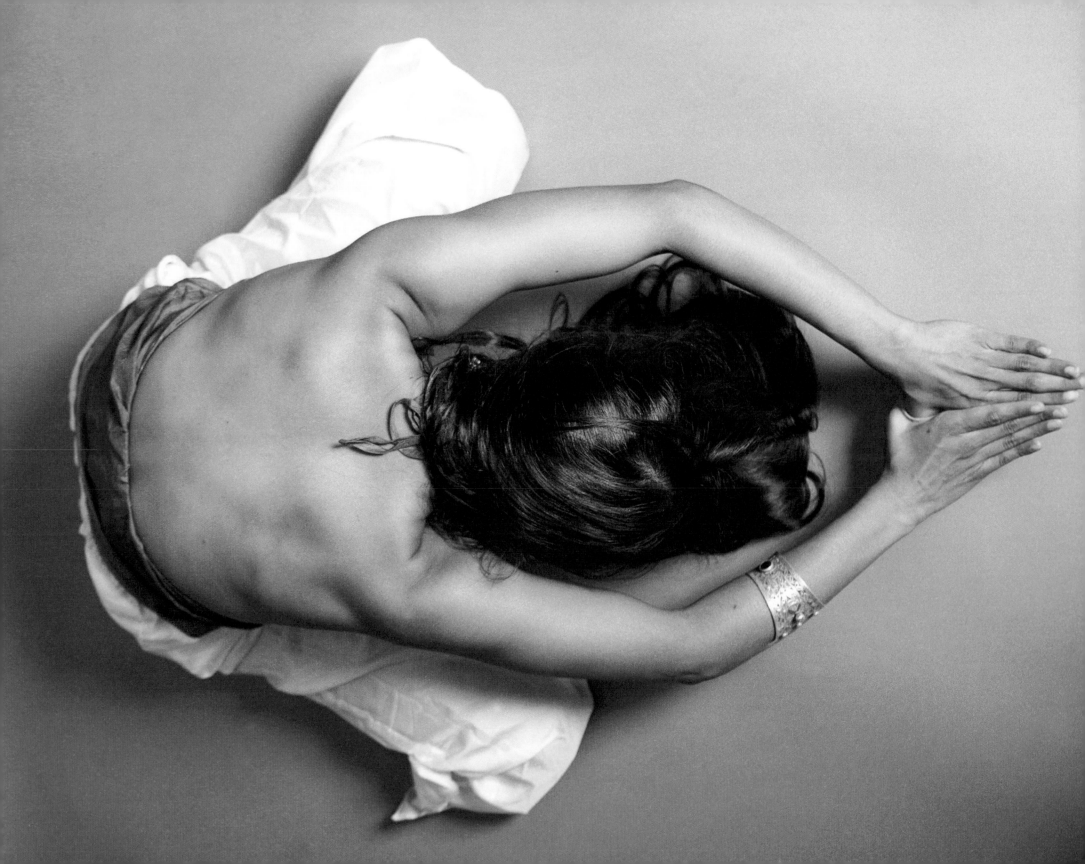

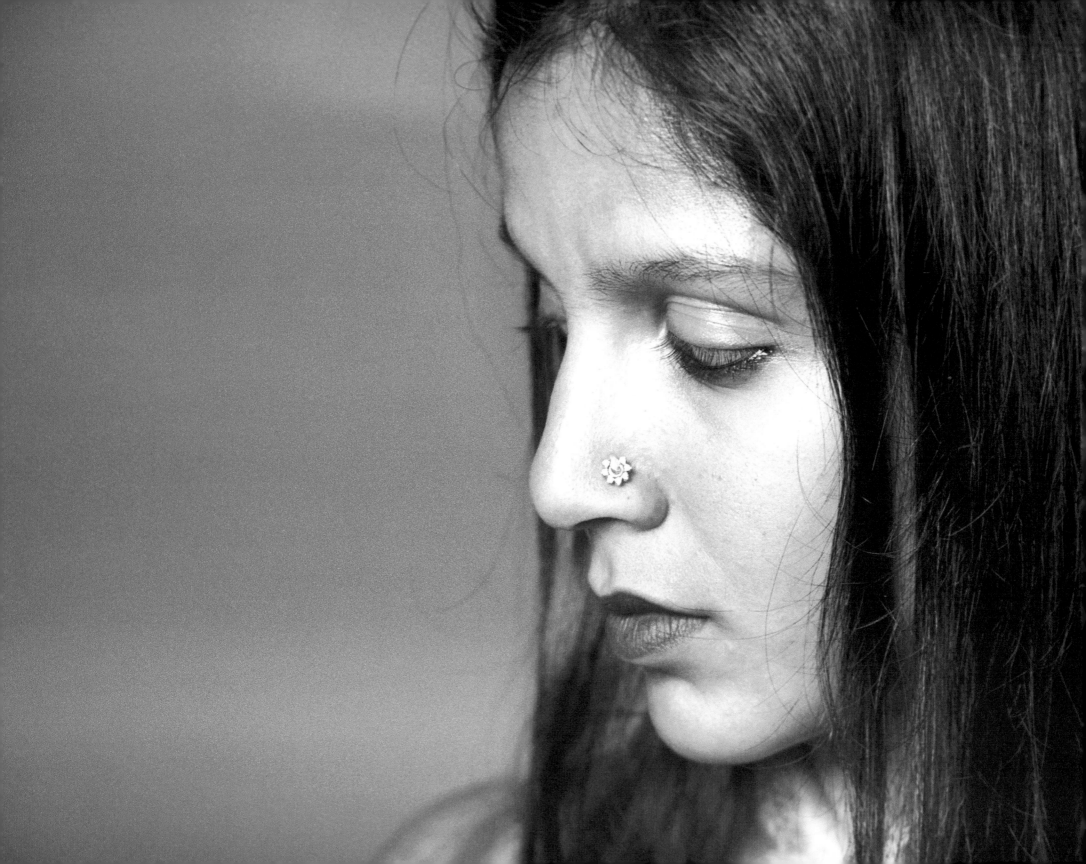

The sun moved in the sky
From the east to the other end.
Fatigued, and perspiring,
he dived into the western ocean for a bath.

ATURKURI MOLLA

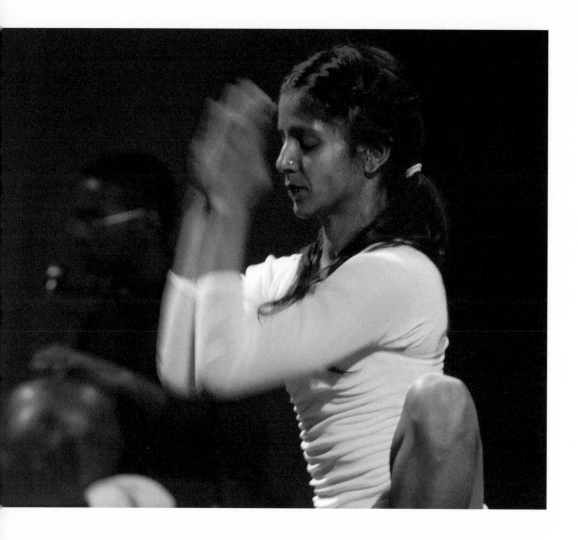

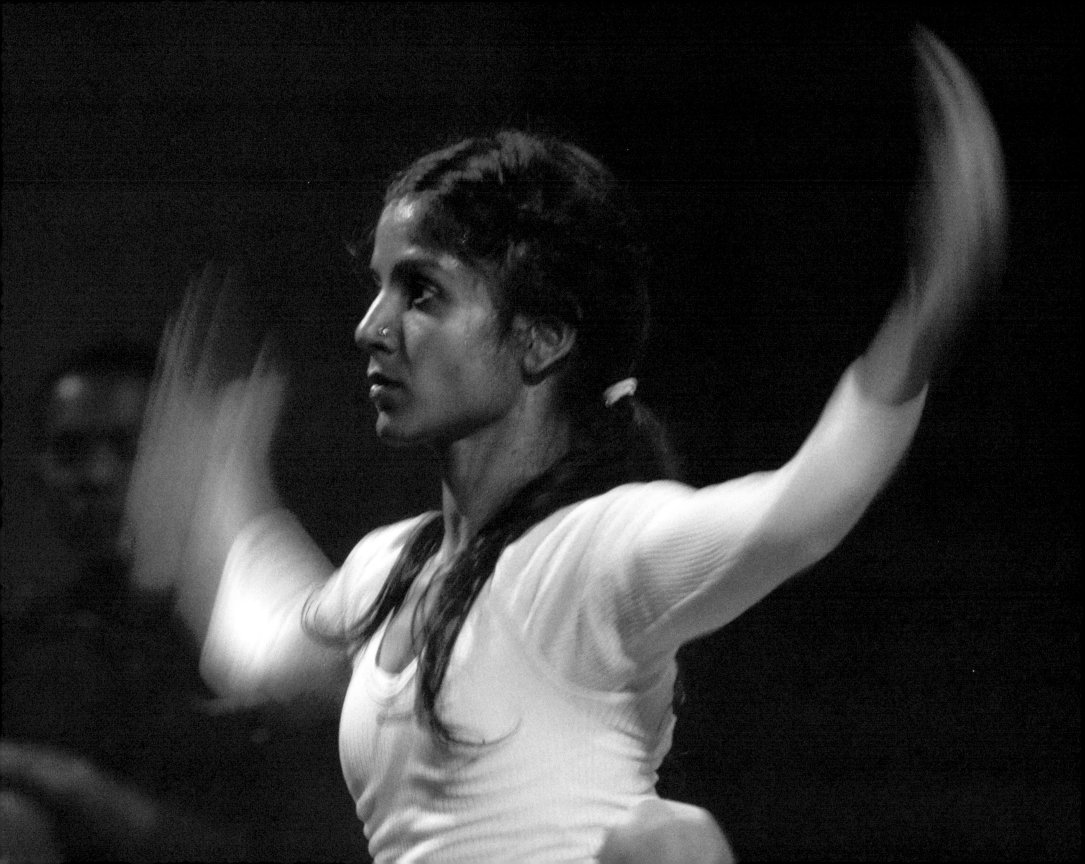

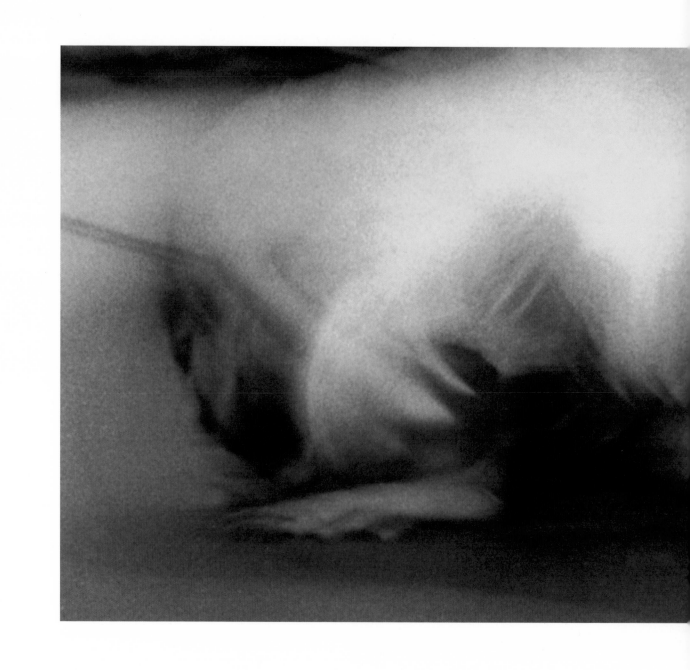

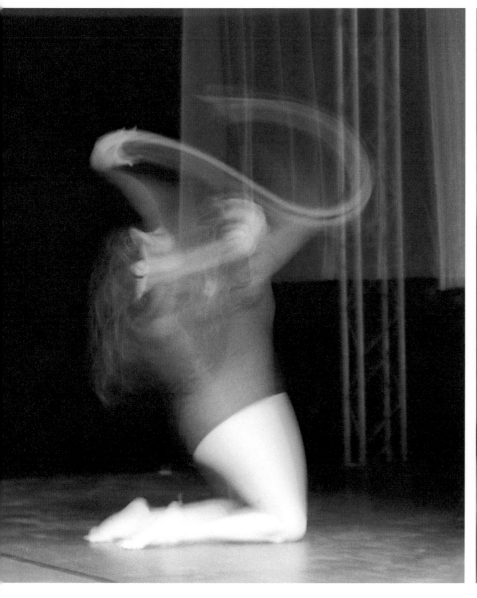
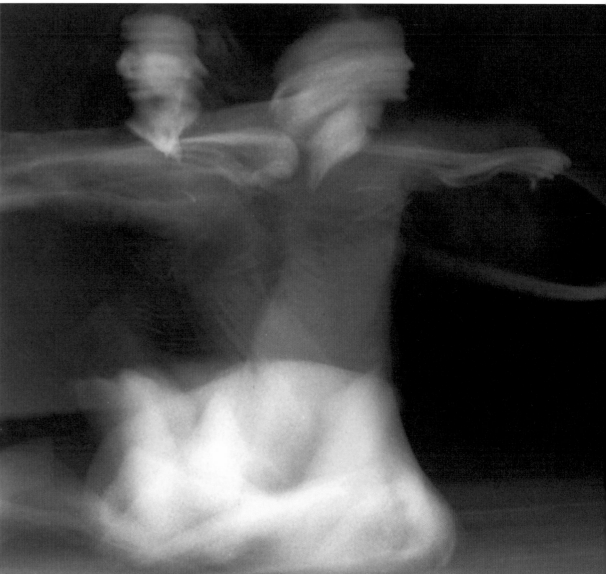

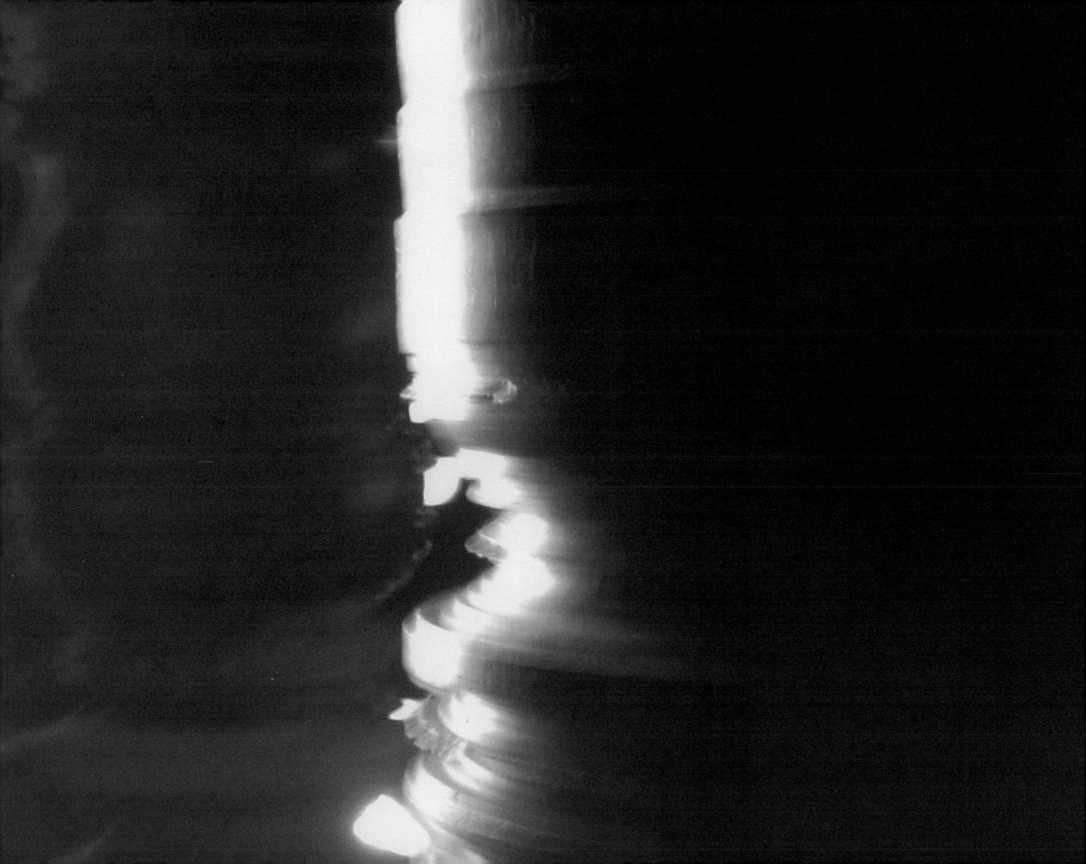

'My eyes drown in the darkness of joy
My heart, like a lotus, closes its petals in the rapture of the dark night.'

VILLAGE MYSTIC POET

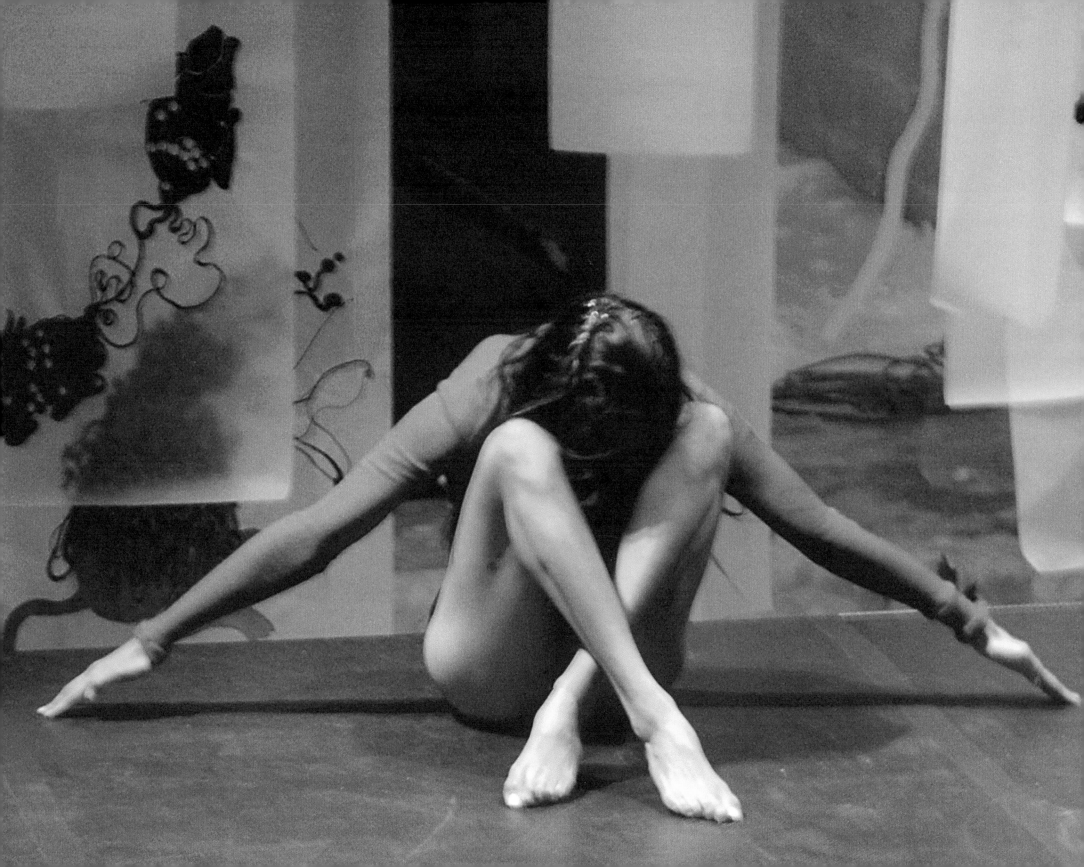

'At first there was only darkness wrapped in darkness.

All this was only unilluminated water.

That One which came to be, enclosed in nothing,

Arose at last, born of the power of heat.'

RG VEDA

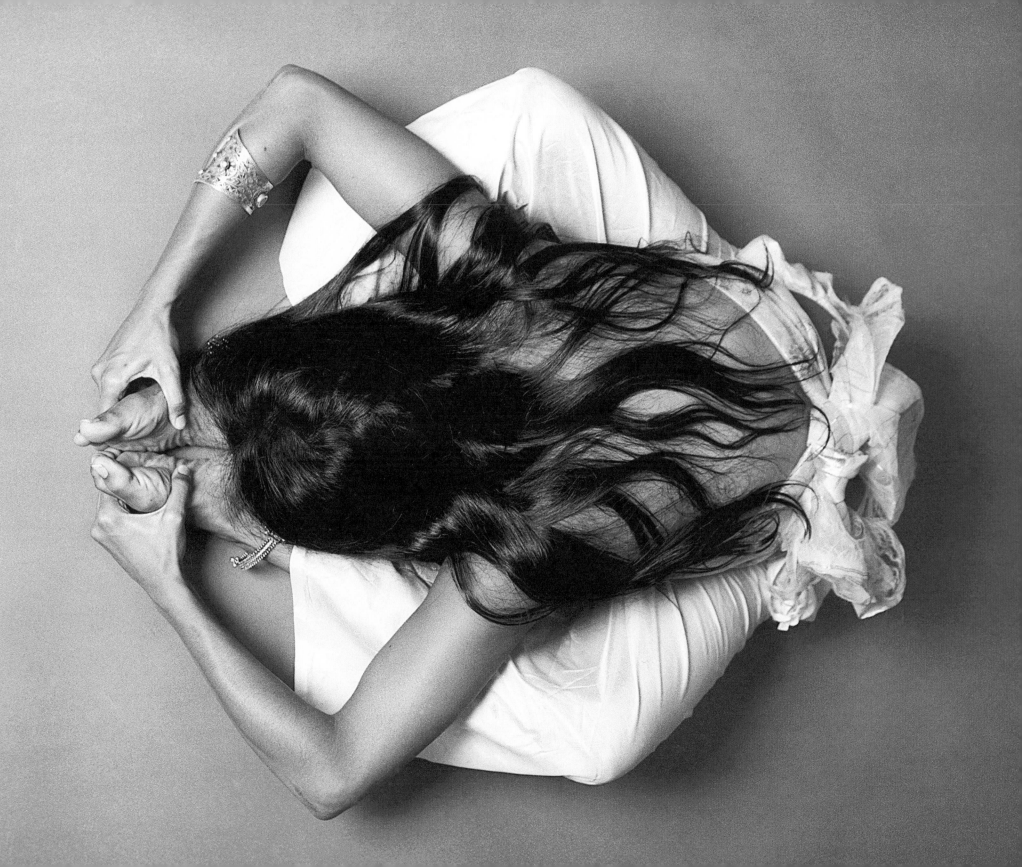

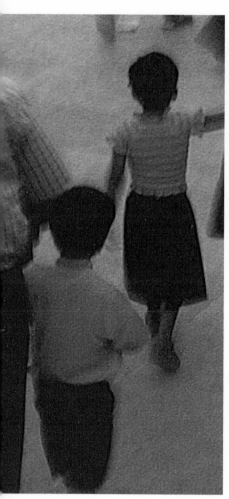
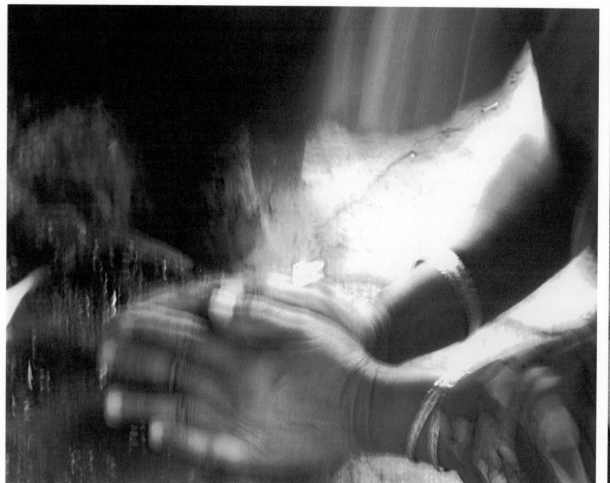
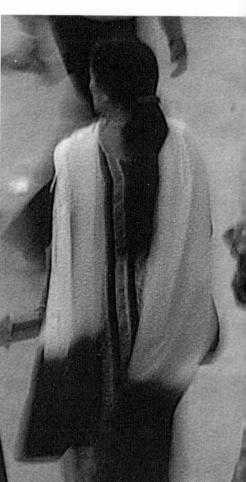

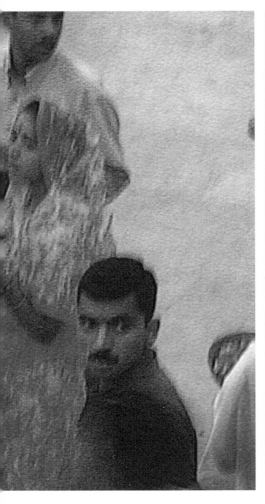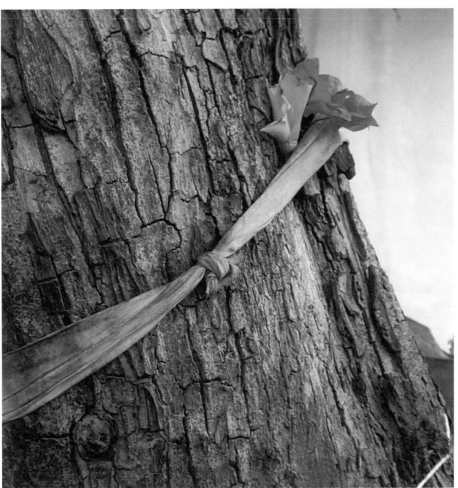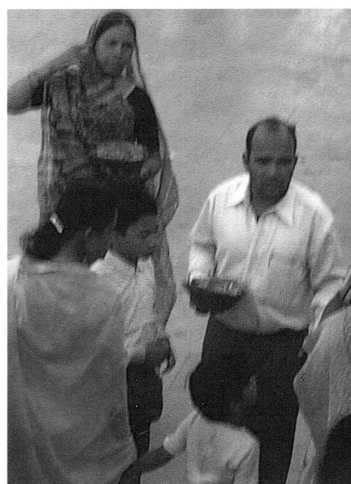

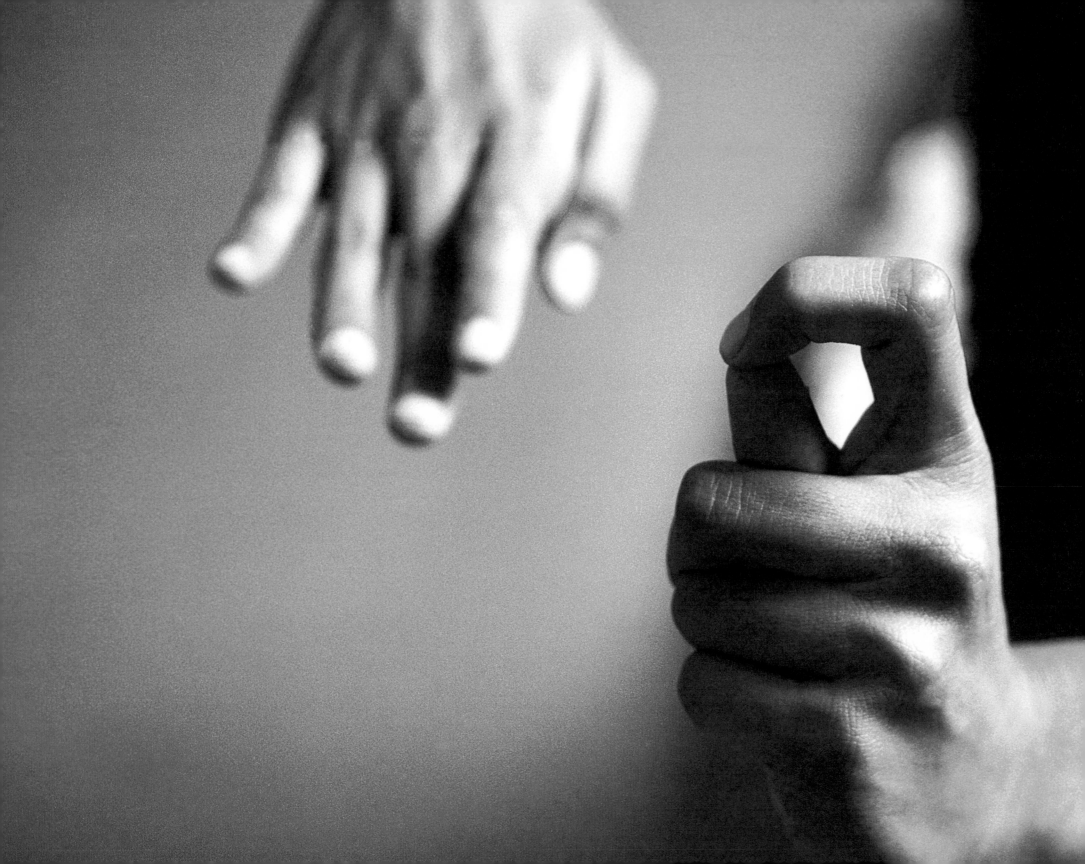

Make thy body the lower fire-stick

[the syllable] Om the upper;

Make use of meditation like the friction [of the sticks],

Then wilt though see God, like hidden [fire]

UPANISHAD

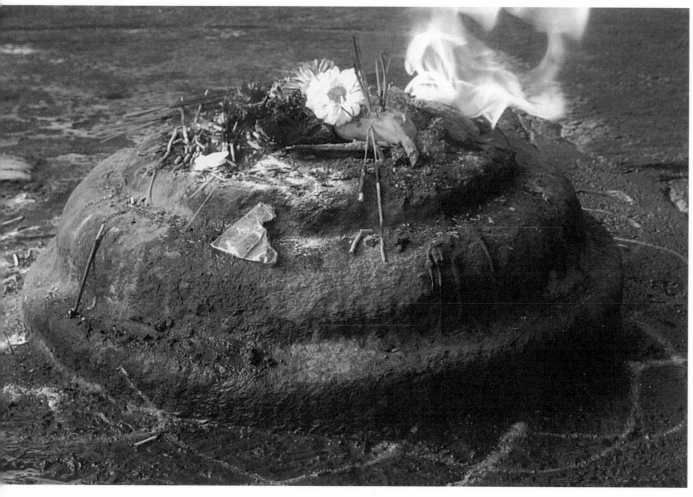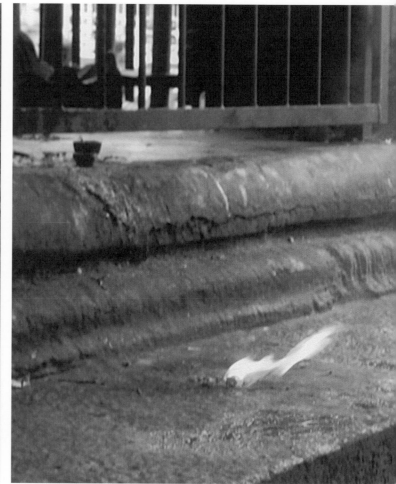

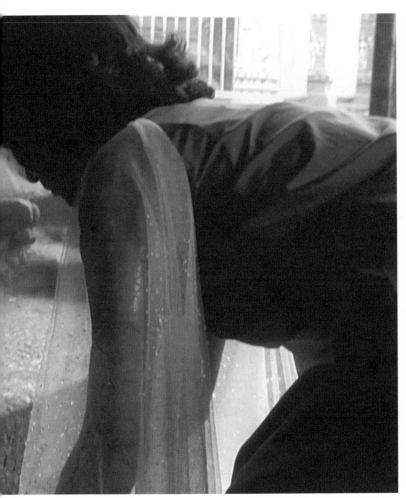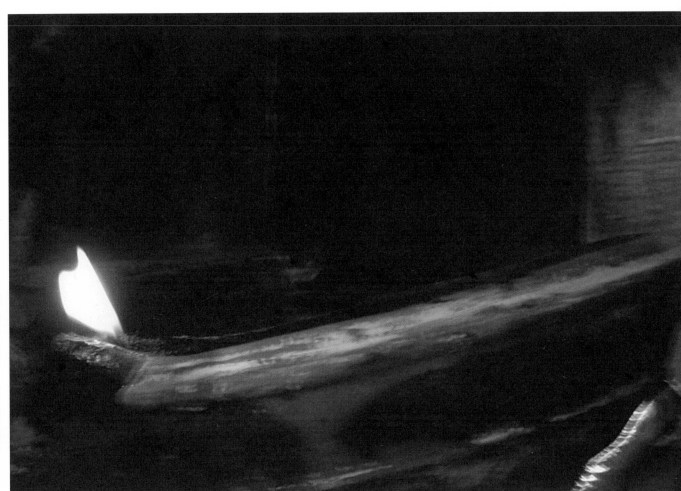

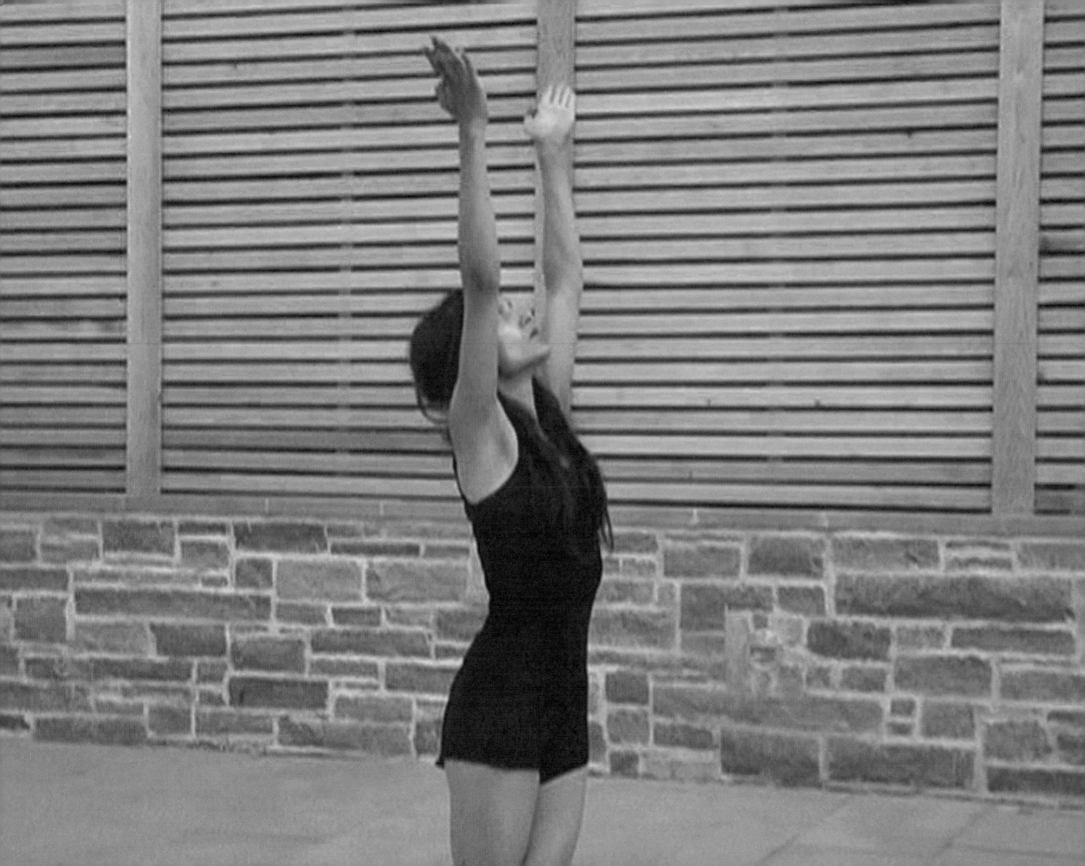

XXI

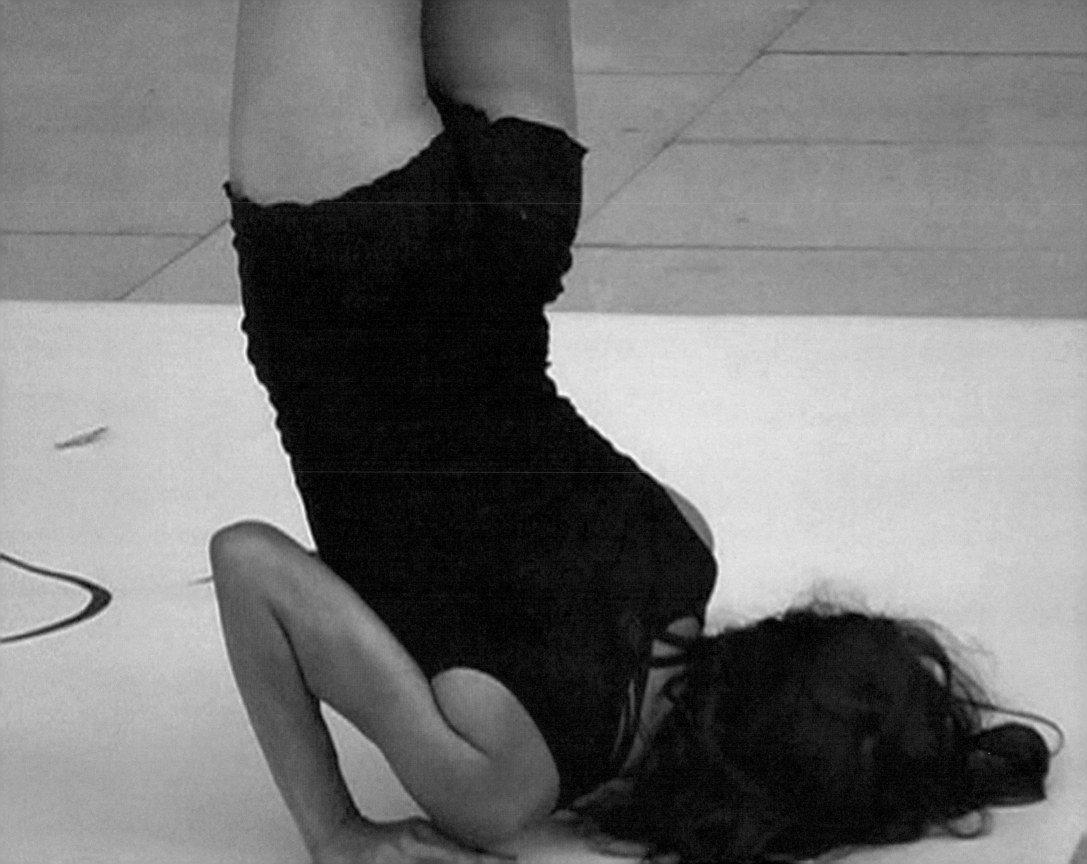

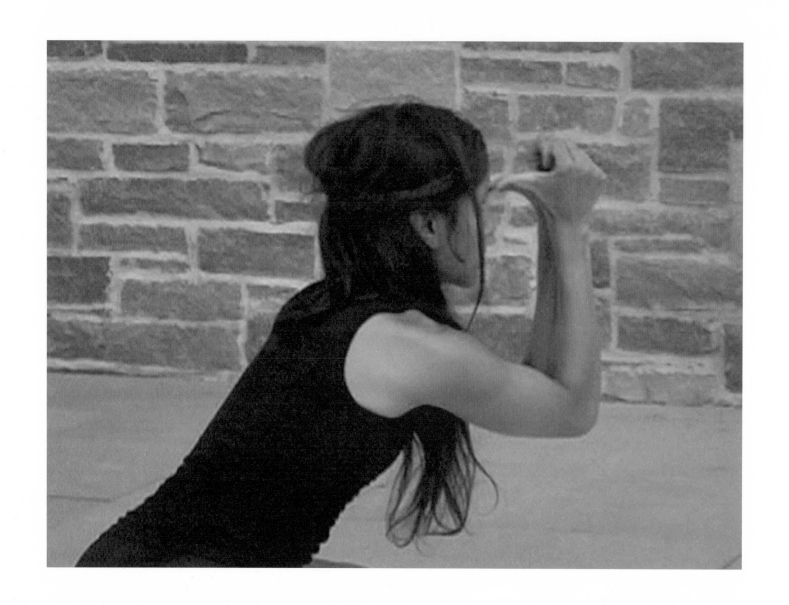

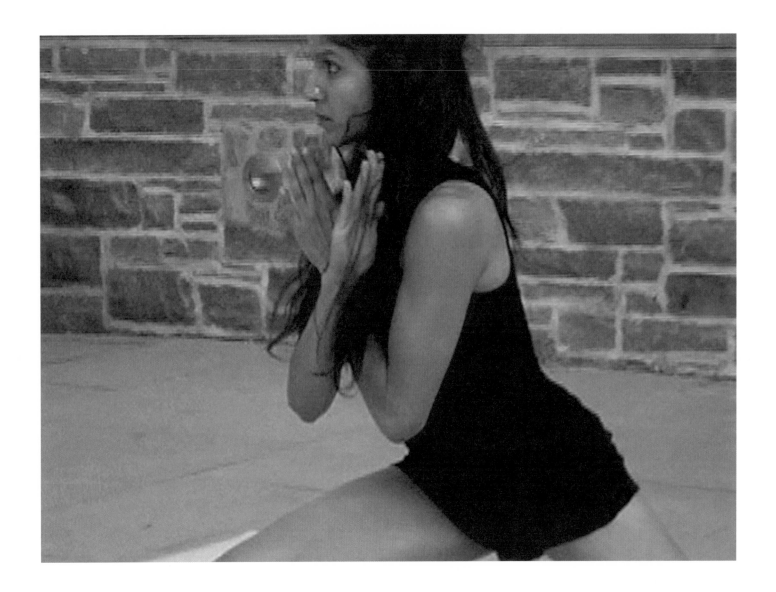

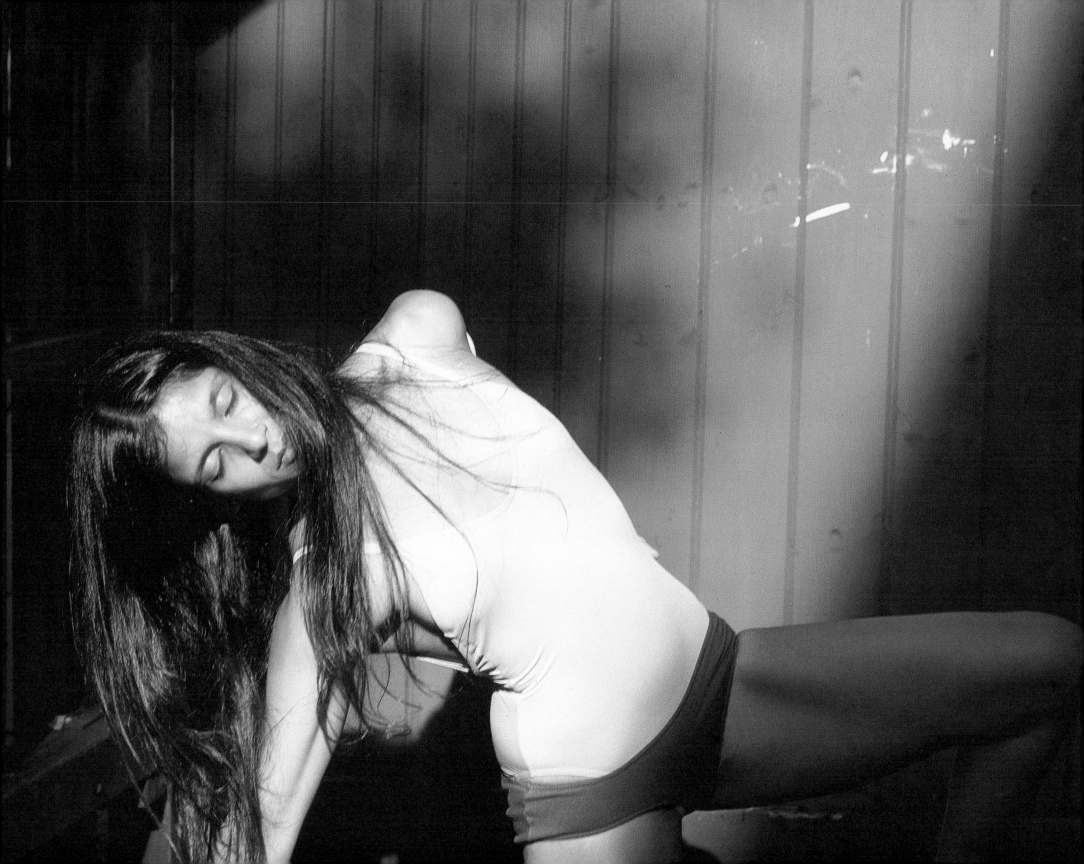

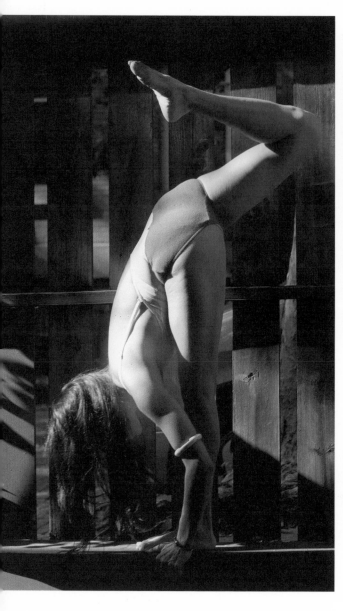

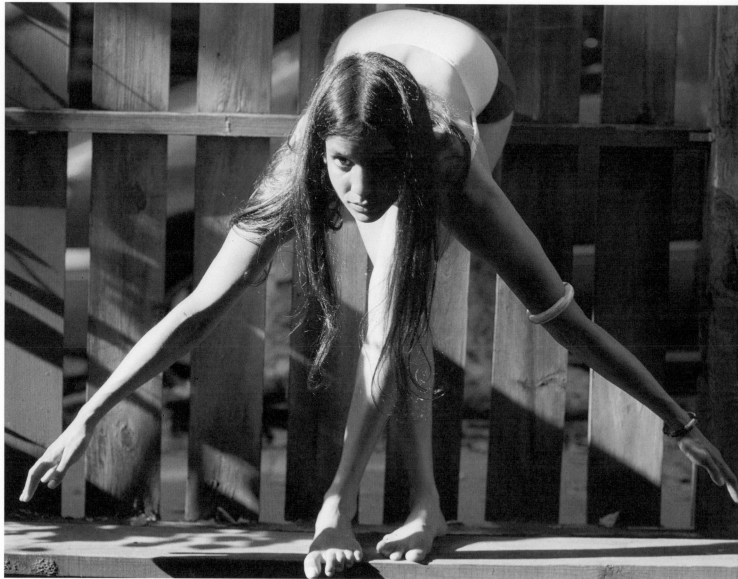

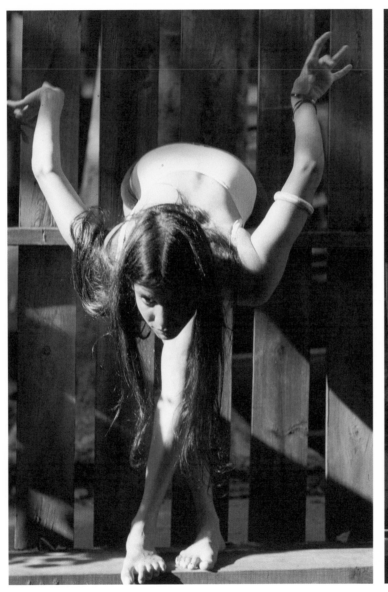
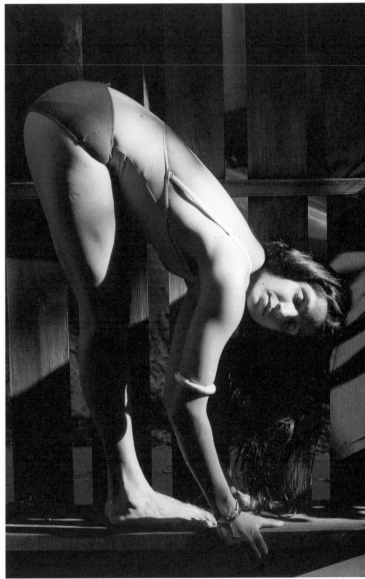

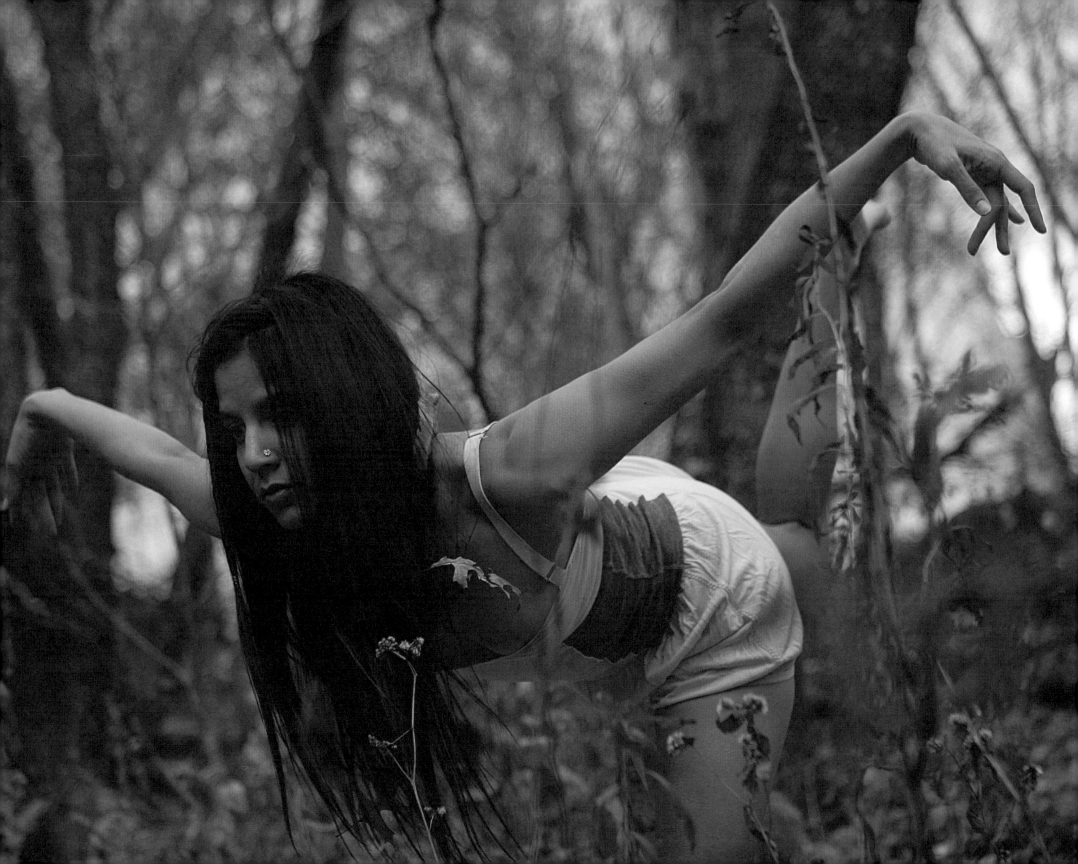

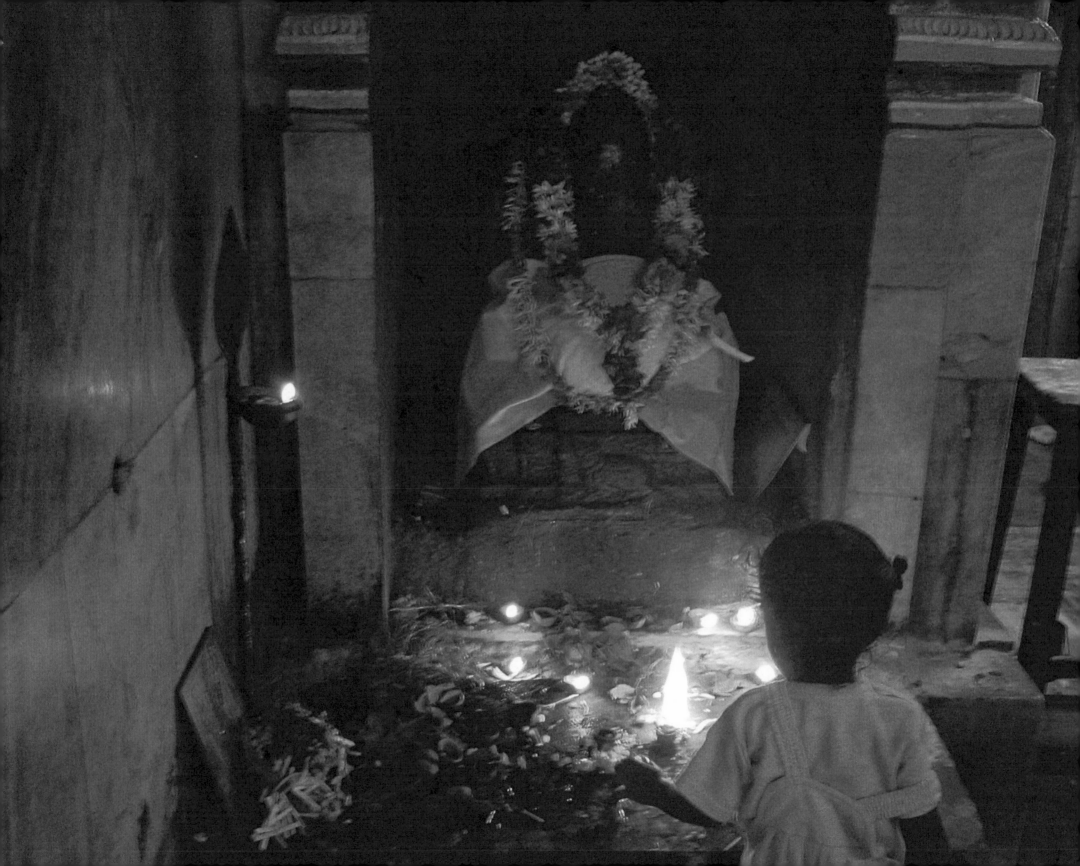

Creative heat, starting a new vibration in the Primal Matter,
gives rise to creative desire,
the will-to-be which acts as the seed of the mind,
the imaginative principle,
and from this follows the entire series of creations of visible,
tangible forms.

NASADIYA SUKTA, RG VEDA

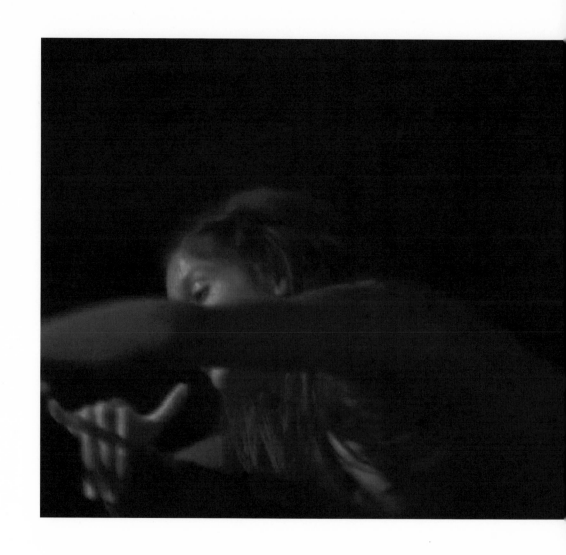

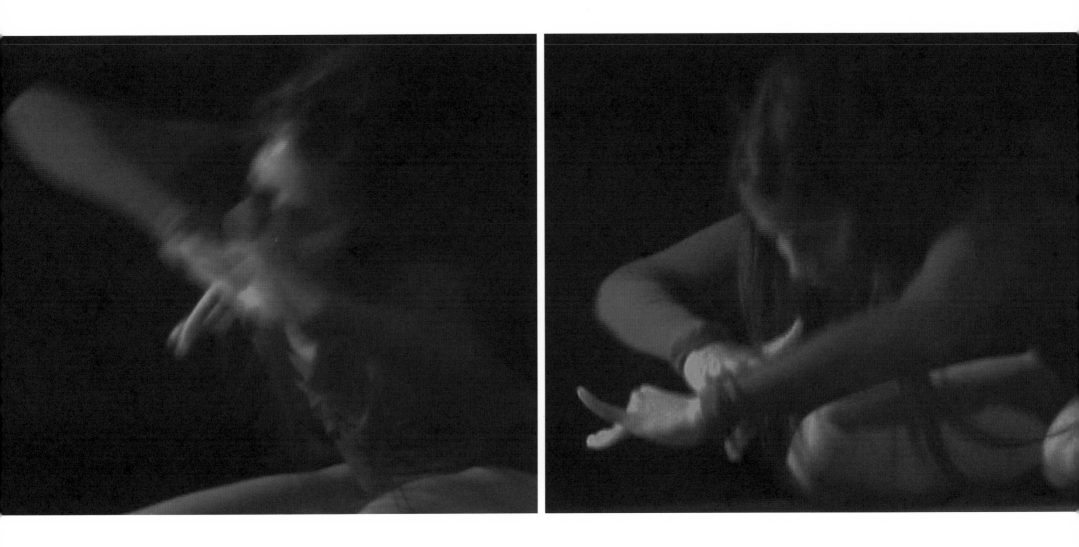

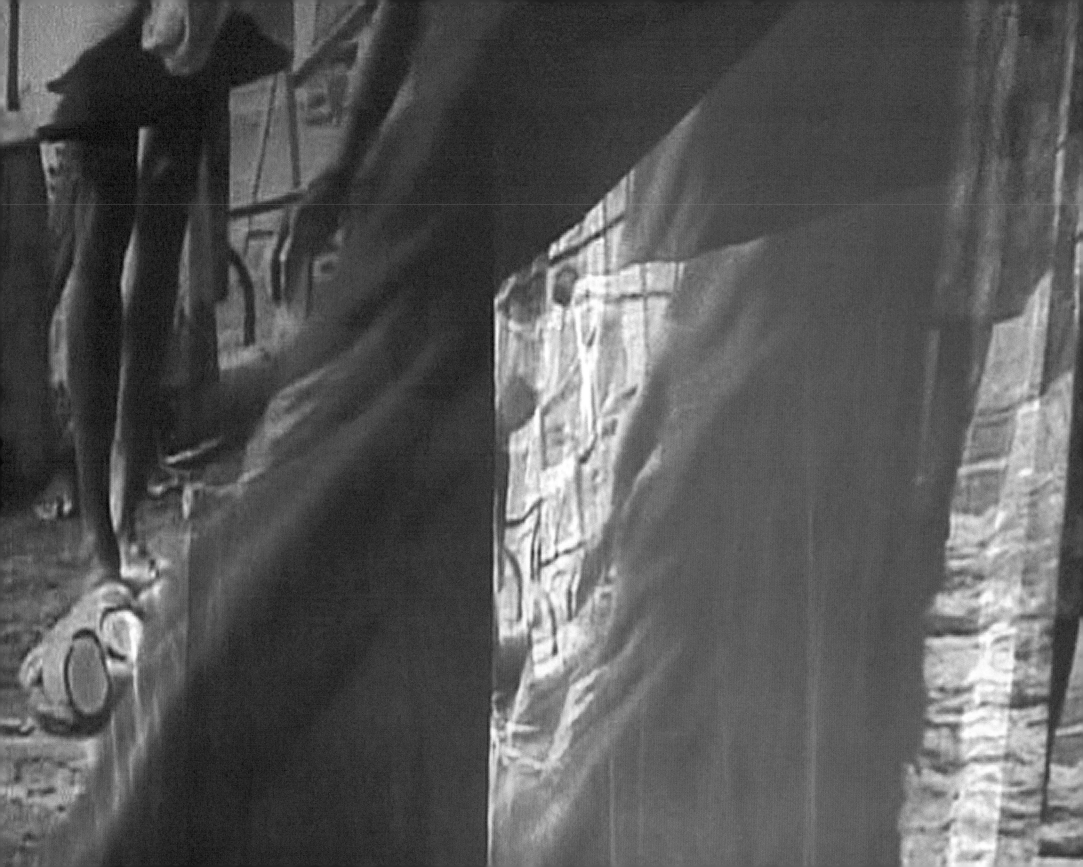

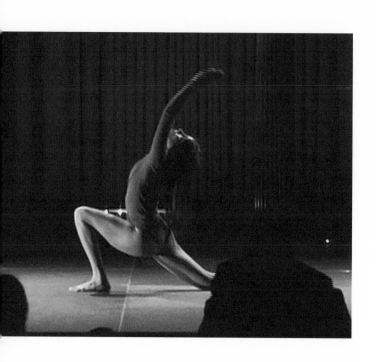
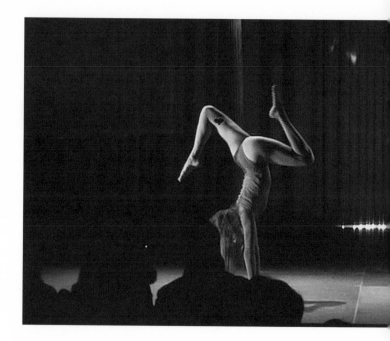

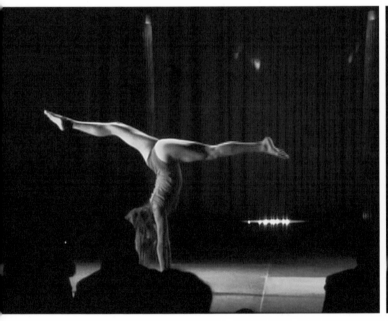 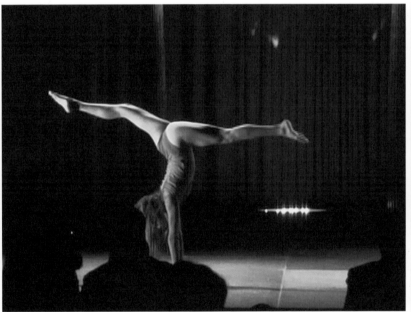 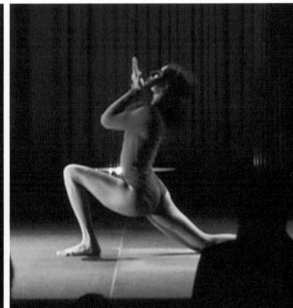

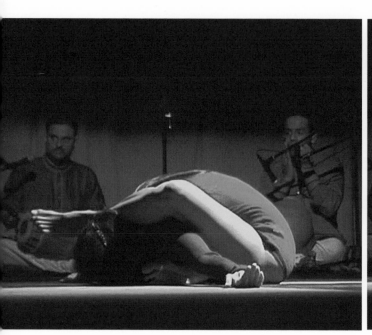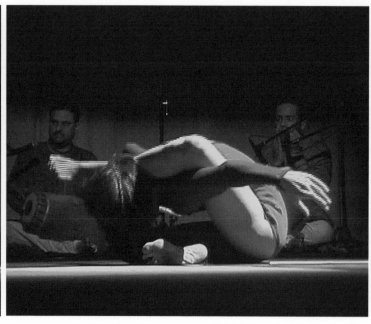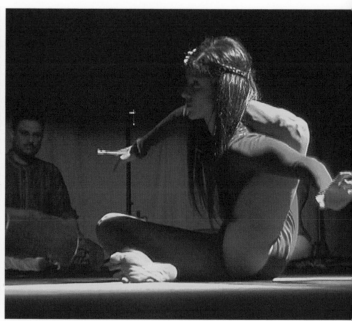

It is the magic of mathematics, the rhythm which is in the heart of all creation, which moves in the atom…. Churn[ing] up images from the vague and makes tangible what is elusive.'

MAHANIRVANA TANTRA

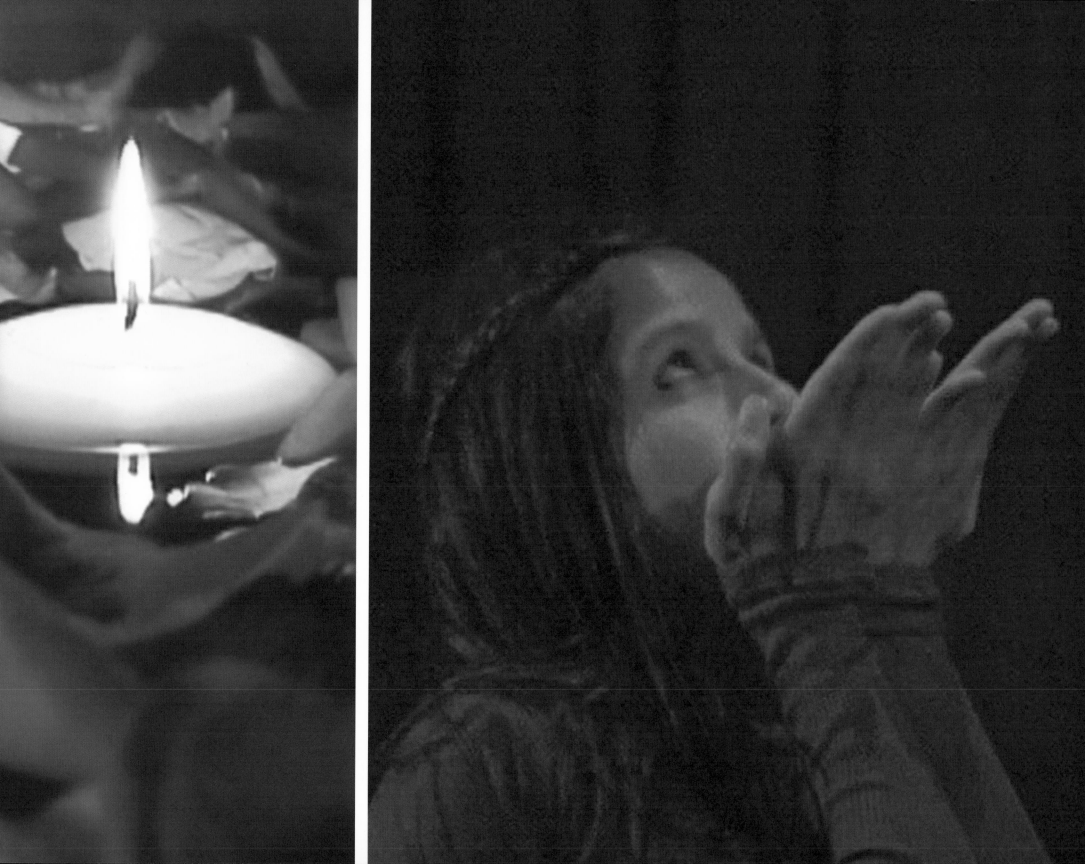

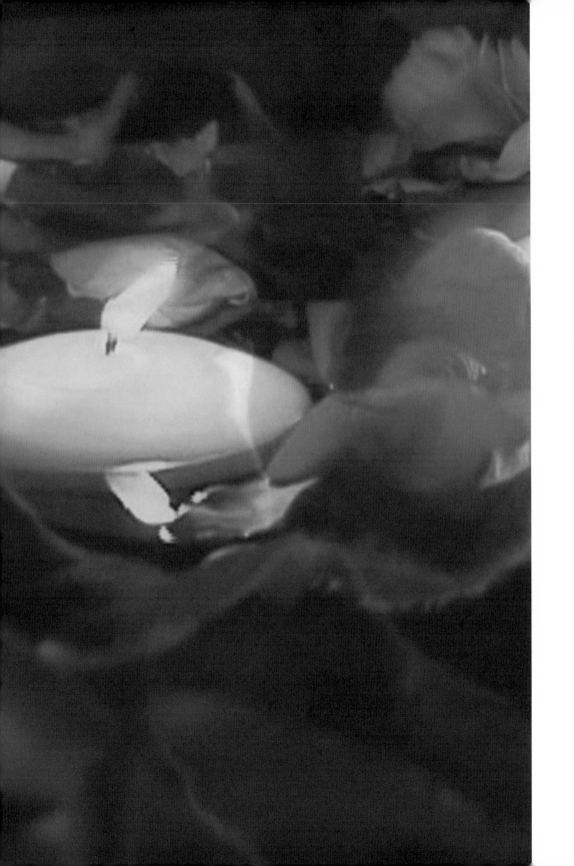

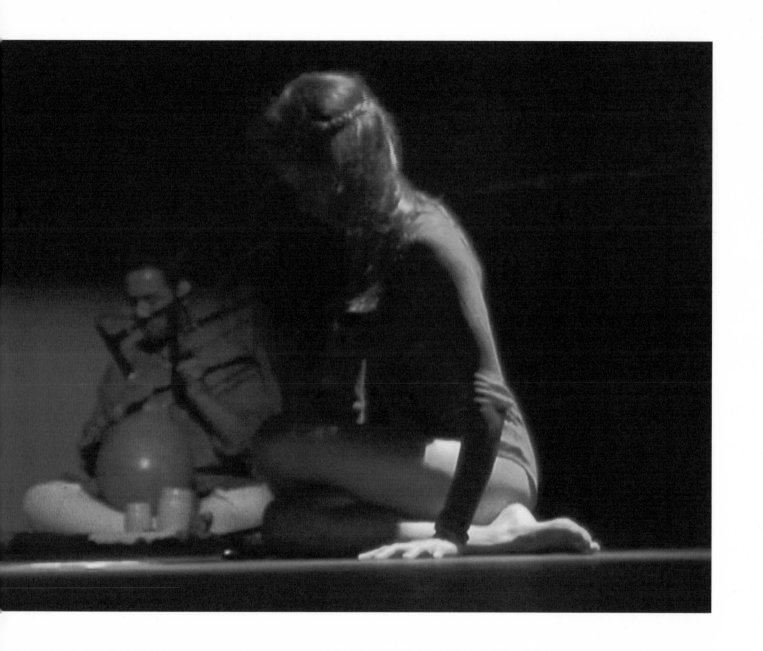

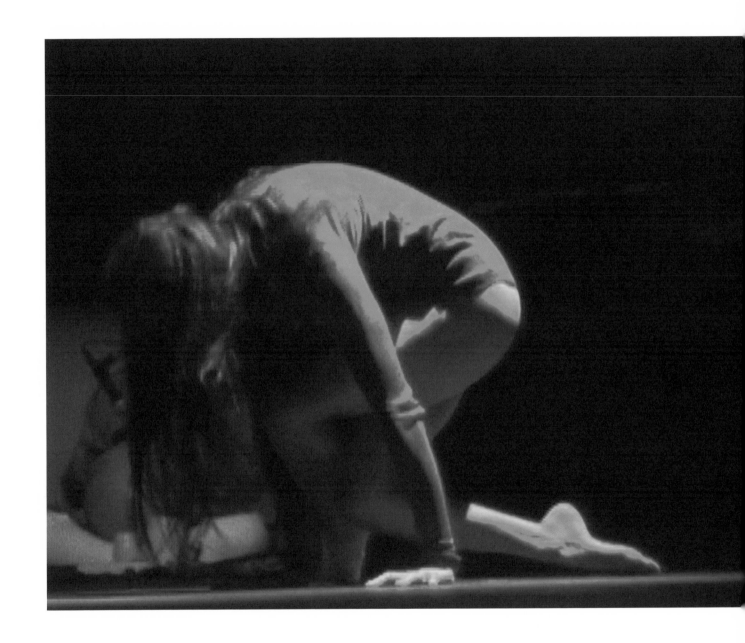

'Everywhere in this earth the paradise is awake and sending forth its voice.
It reaches our inner ear without knowing it… It tunes our harp of life… not only
in prayers and hopes, but also…in the dance which is the ecstatic meditation
in the still centre of movement.'

RABINDRANATH TAGORE

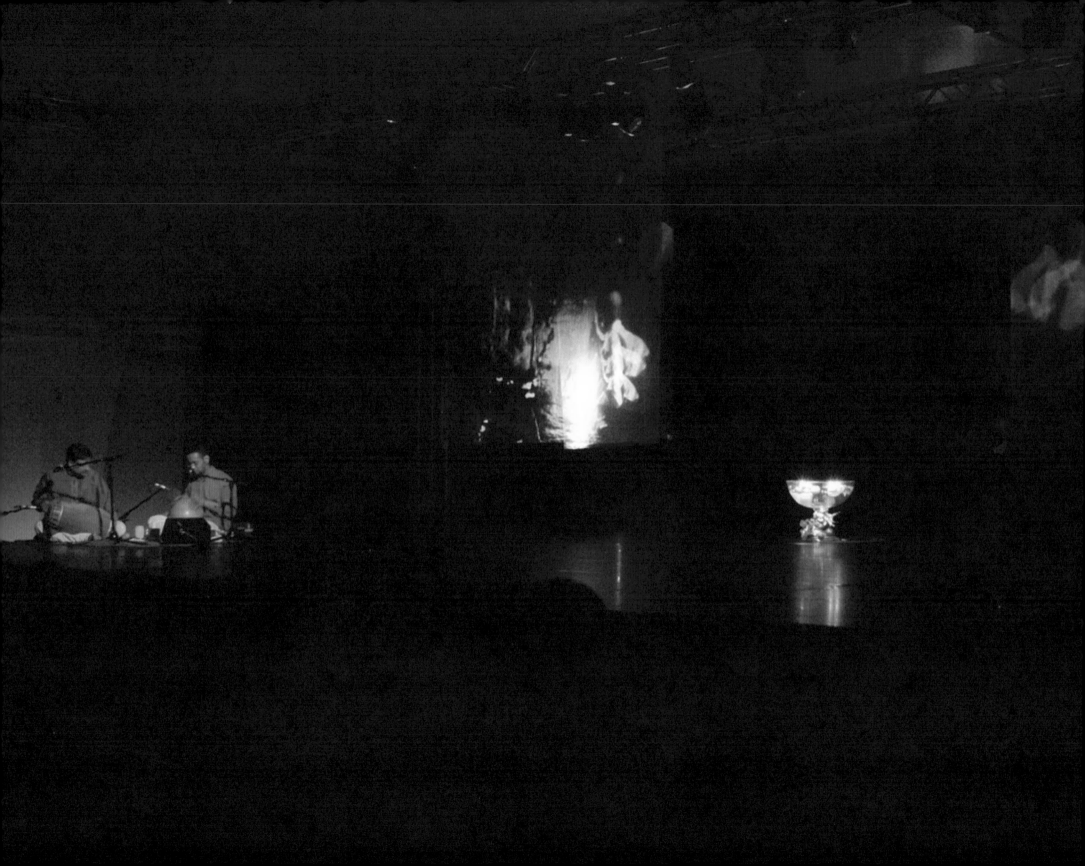

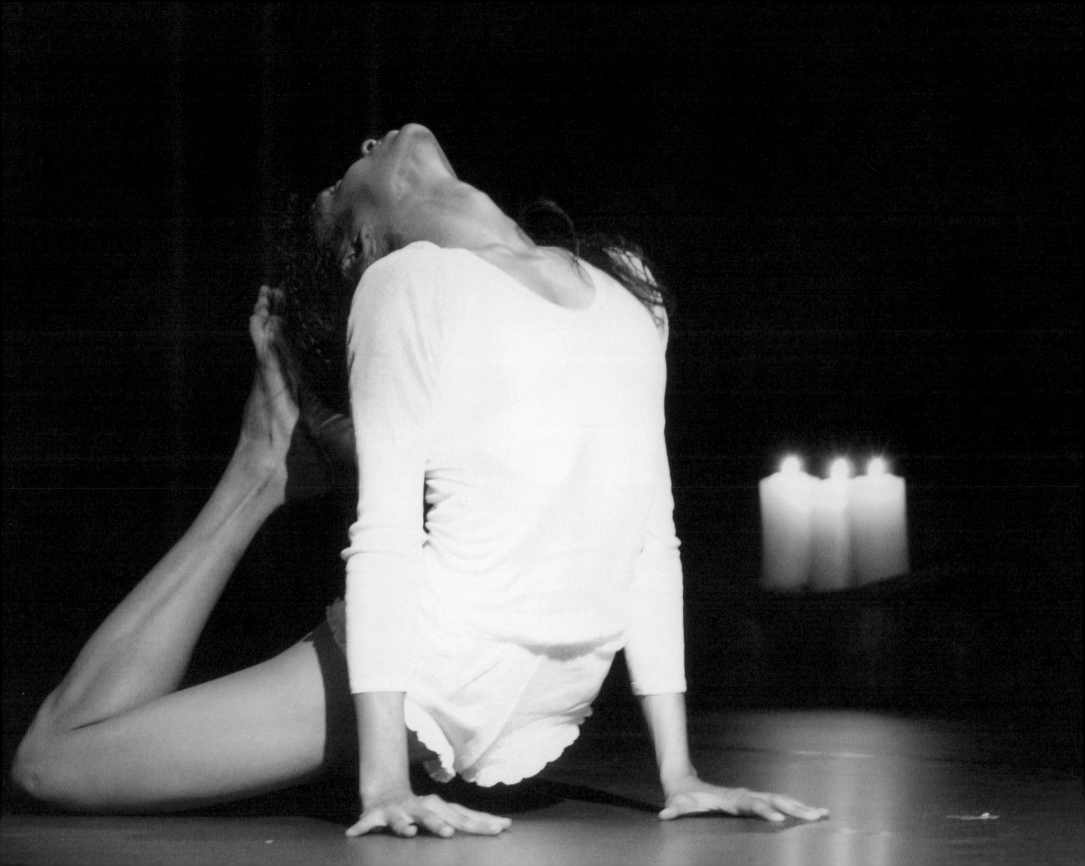

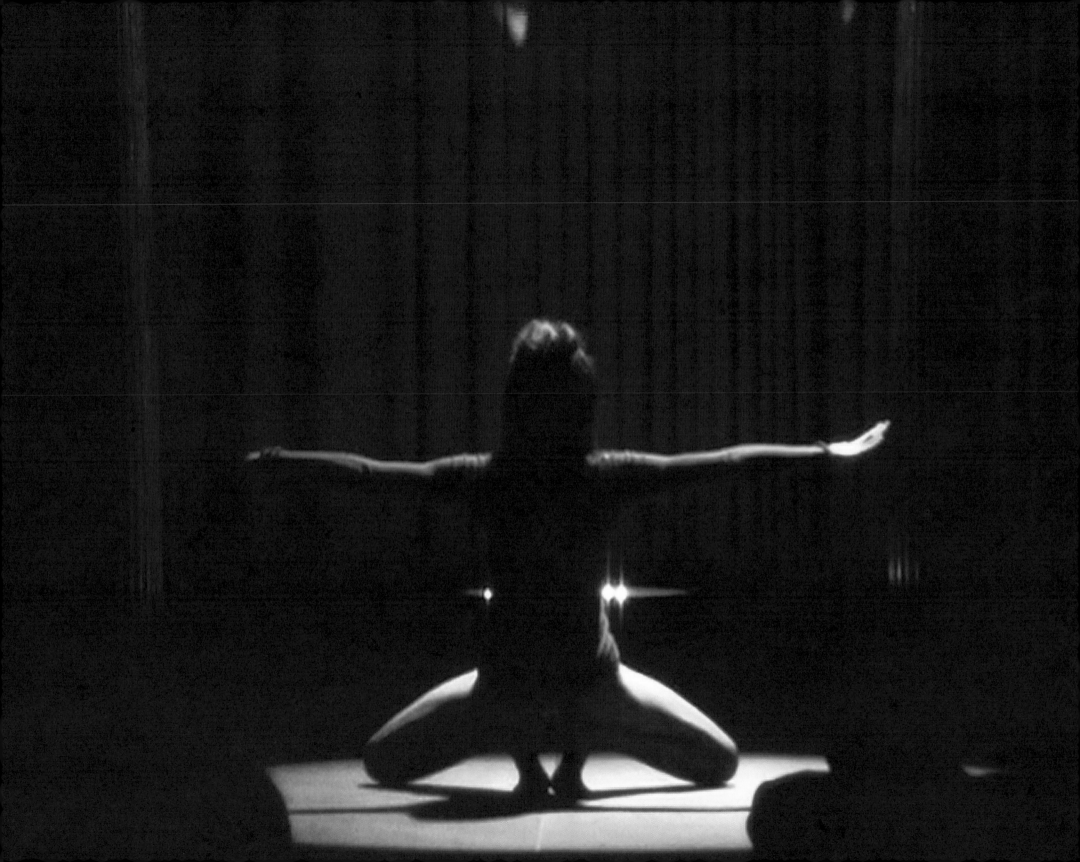

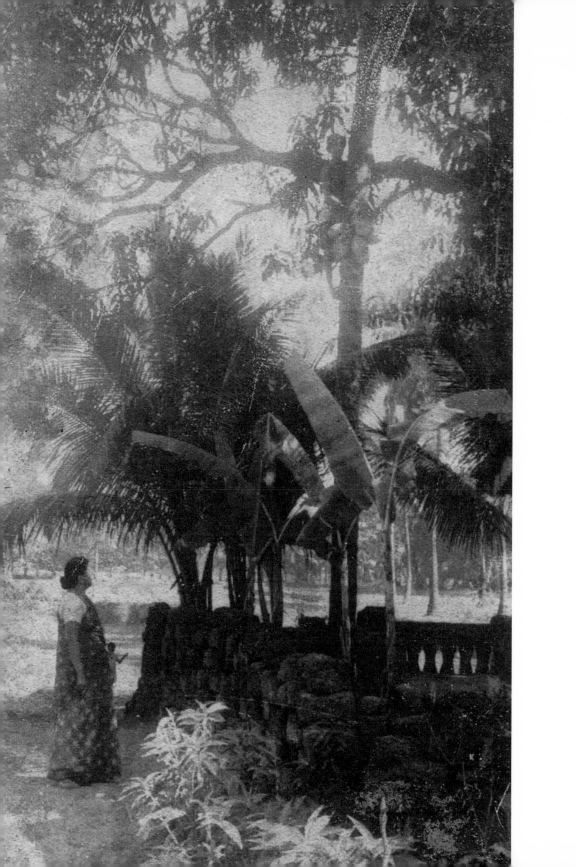

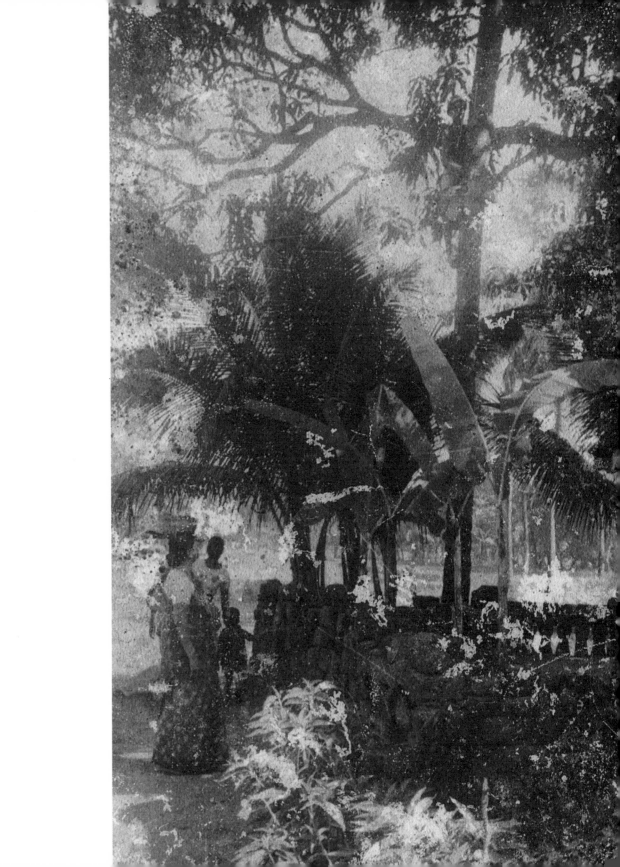

Let a man revere [the sun] up there which radiates heat as the syllable Om;
For on rising it sings aloud for the sake of [all] creatures'

CHANDOGYA UPANISHAD

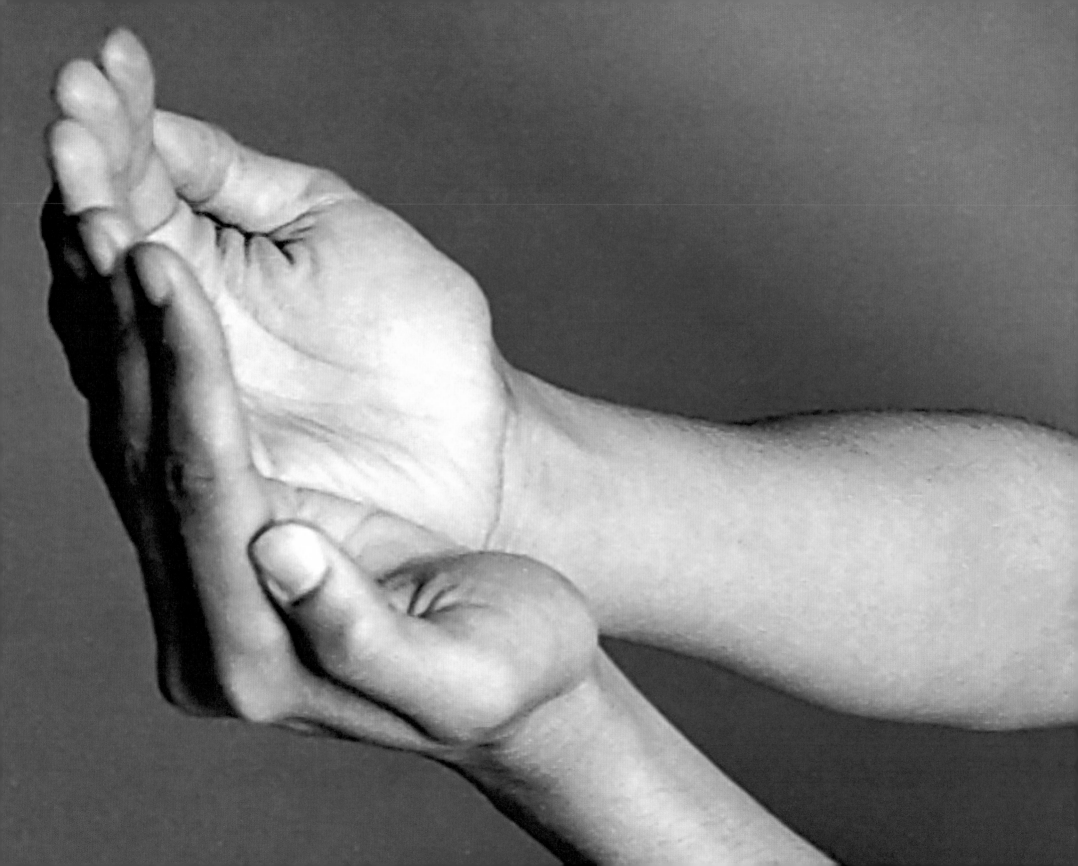

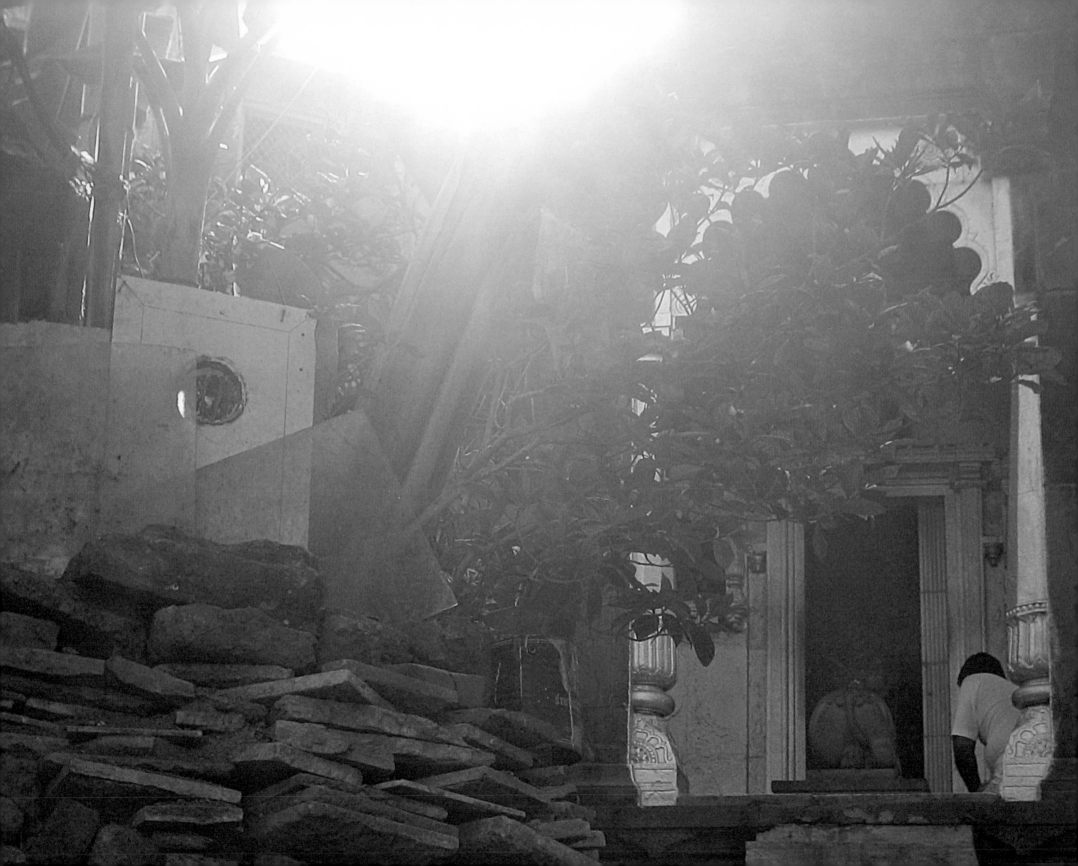

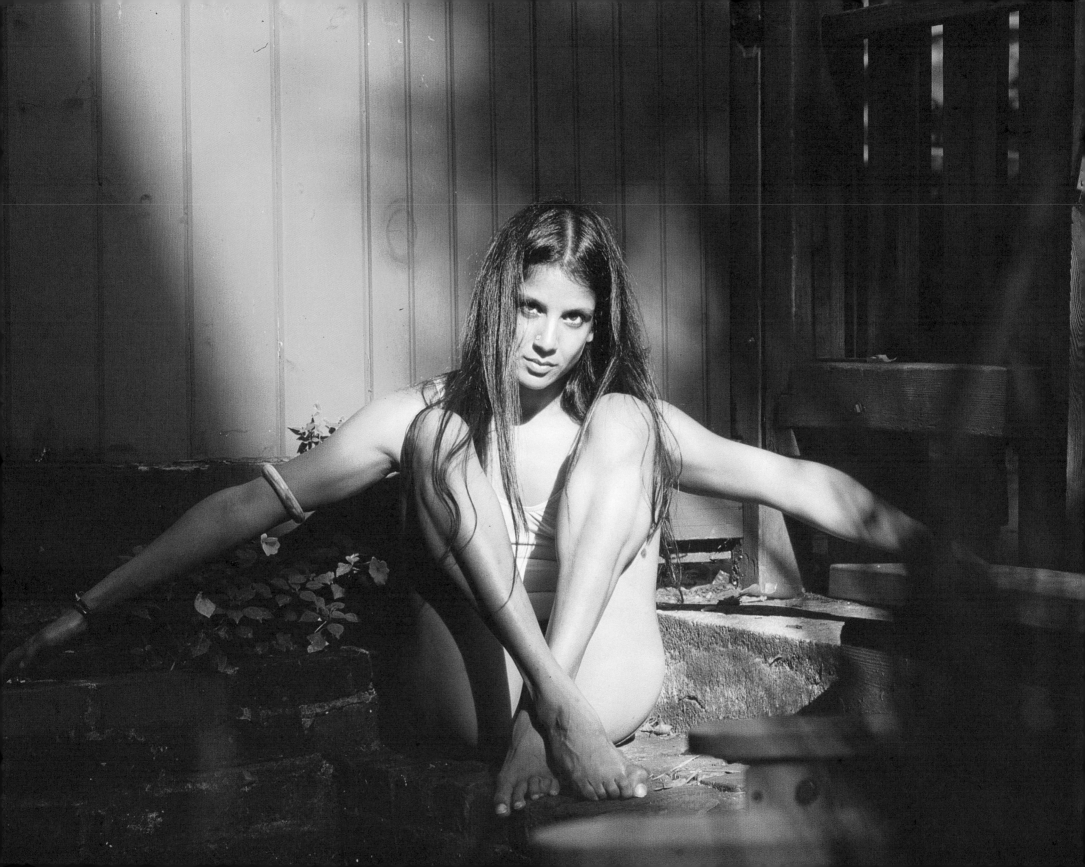

At the day's dawning all things manifest
Spring forth from the Unmanifest.

BHAGAVAD GITA

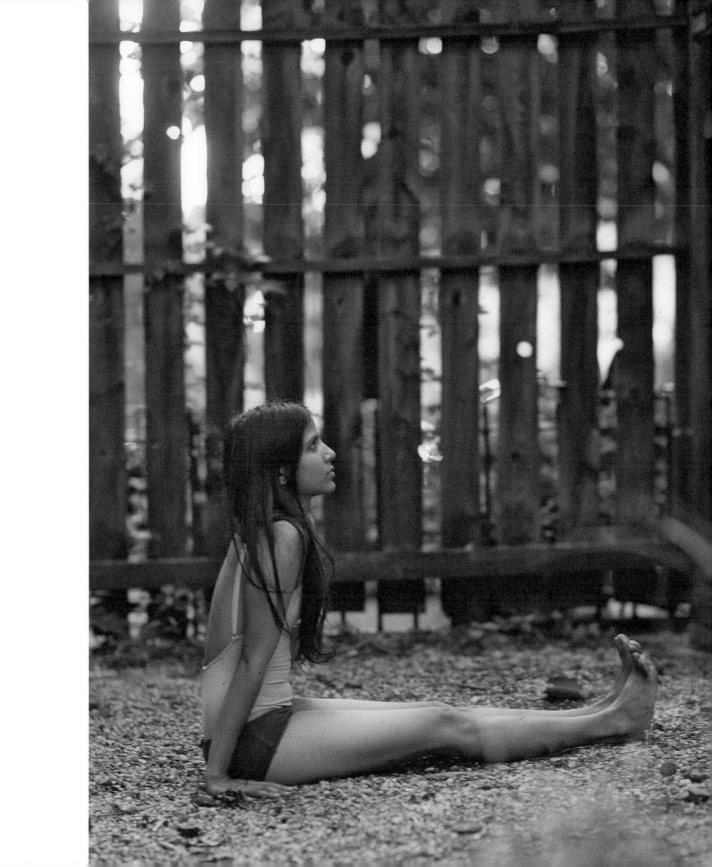

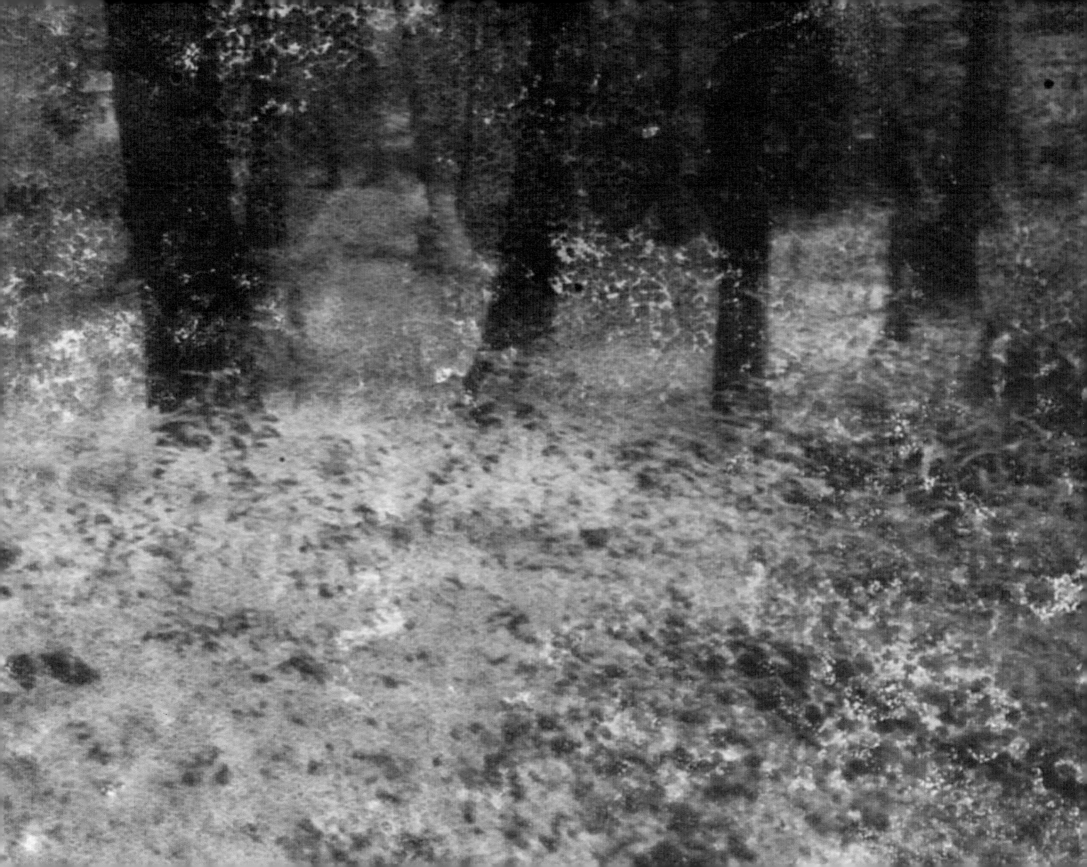

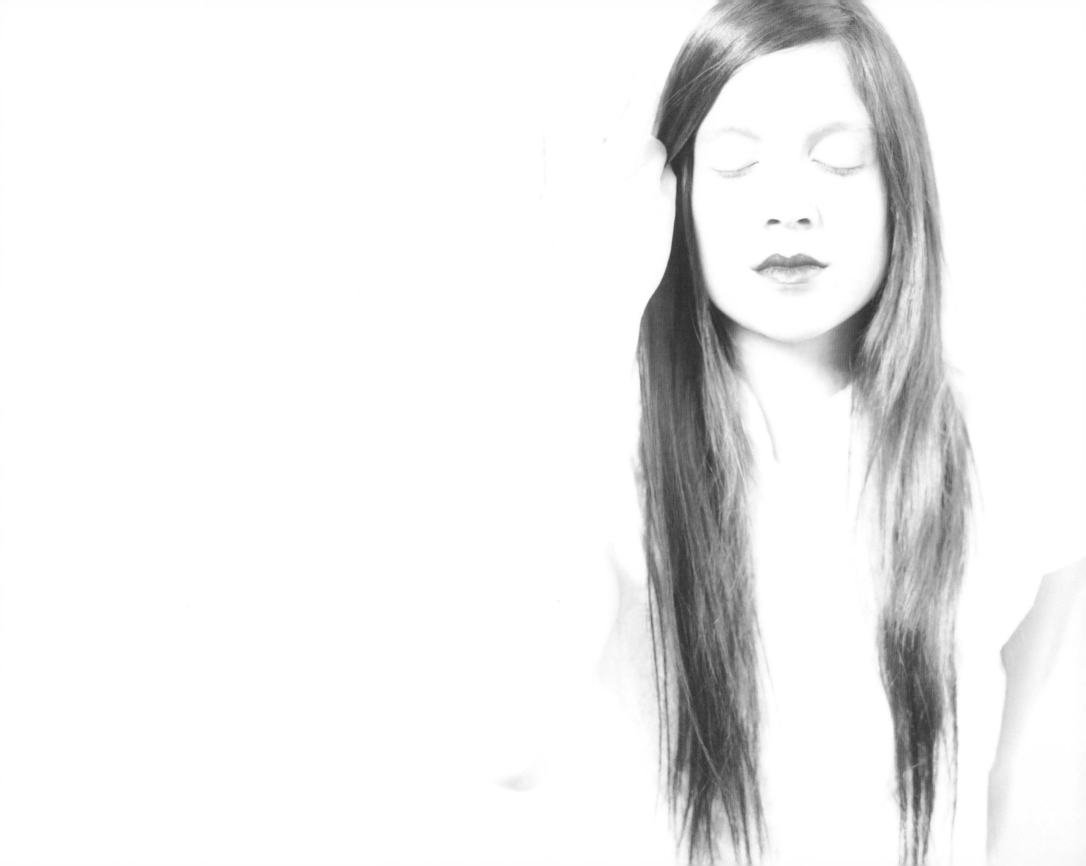

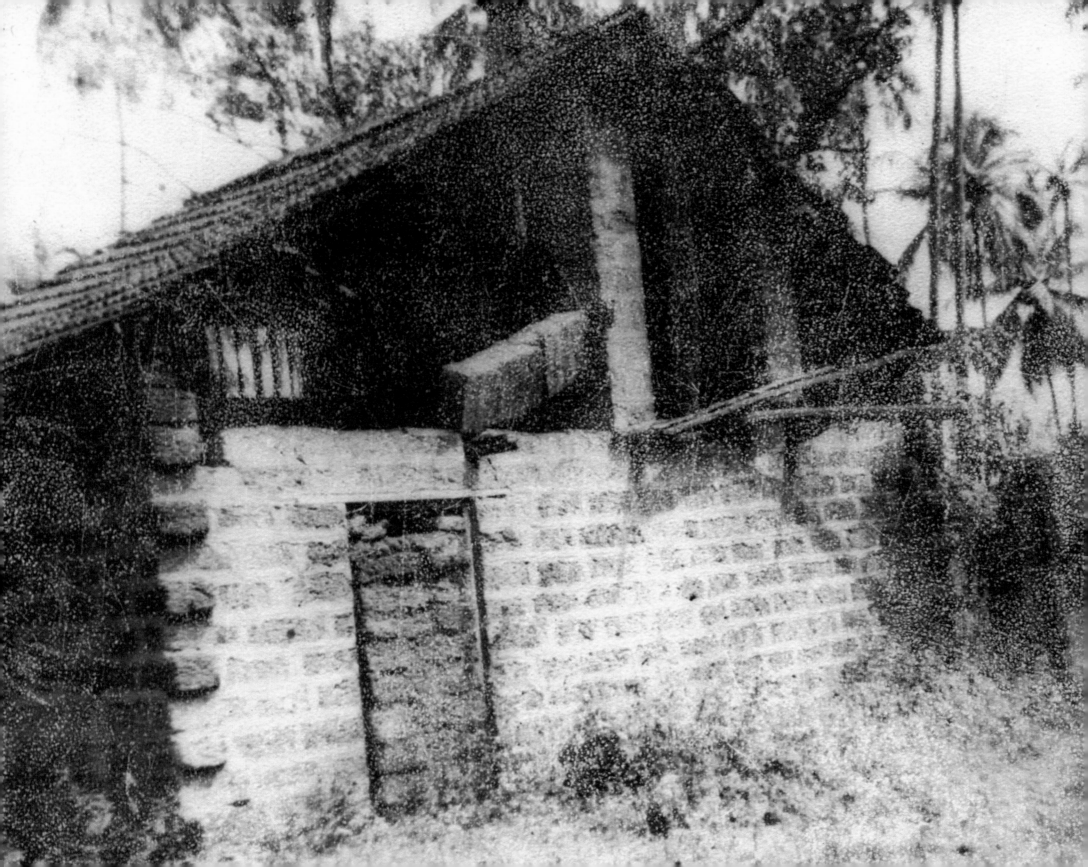

SHARMILA, THE LIVING SCULPTURE

On a visit to Shahzia Sikander's studio several years ago, I became intrigued by a series of arresting figurative images. In a new group of paintings, Shahzia portrayed a woman in poses I had never before imagined. The body was upside down with the legs gesturing as if they were arms. The torso swiveled in a way that seemed impossible yet looked effortless. Shahzia saw my fascination and said, 'Oh, that's Sharmila.' She then retrieved a portfolio of photographs of a young woman posing on the studio floor, actually engaged in the seemingly impossible poses reproduced in the paintings.

Who was this astonishing model whose poses were like fantastic Hindu sculptures turned upside down? This was my first introduction to Sharmila Desai, who seemed to me like a living sculpture. Shahzia had seen Sharmila perform and invited her to collaborate on a series of paintings. Intrigued, I asked Shahzia to take me along to Sharmila's next performance.

Just as Shahzia Sikander has created an unexpected mixture of traditional and modern, Eastern and Western in her painting, Sharmila Desai has also created a strikingly original fusion, combining rigorous yoga practice with traditional Indian dance and modern dance. I first witnessed her in action as part of an otherwise raucous evening of short acts by South Asian woman comedians and assorted performance artists. Sharmila stunned the audience into silence. We watched in awe as she performed her entire set standing on her head.

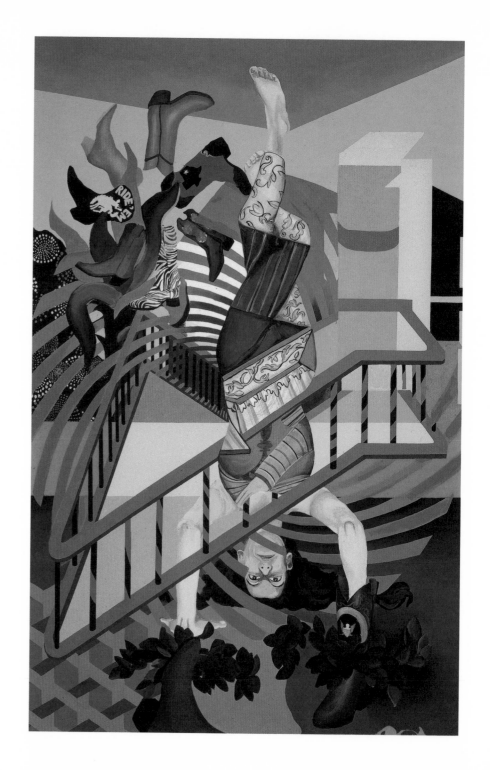

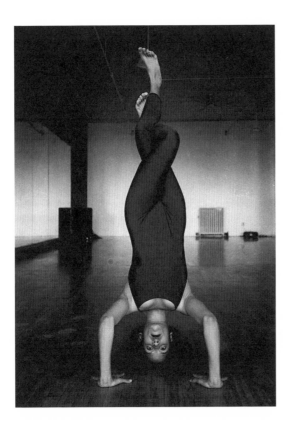

When I become especially excited about someone who is creating a new type of form, I ask them to present a project at our gallery. I asked Sharmila to develop a project for us without specifying whether it should involve dance, music, or sculpture. It turned out to be a remarkable mixture of all three. Her performance was absorbing and inspiring, an invitation to enter Sharmila's unique spiritual and aesthetic world. Entitled *Anjali* 'the *mudra* in which the hands are joined together in prayer form' it conveyed a spirit of ecstatic offering when it was first performed in SoHo in 2004.

While presenting Sharmila's project I was fascinated, but not really surprised to find out that Sharmila had developed collaborative relationships with a circle of art historians, choreographers, actors, artists and musicians, several of whom were also doing projects with the gallery. Sharmila was inspiring people from a range of creative disciplines to expand the possibilities of their form.

One of the most important innovations in visual art during the past decade has been the mixing of forms: traditional meets contemporary, Western meets non-Western. Like a DJs smash-up of Bollywood and hip-hop, or punk with Japanese pop, unanticipated combinations have created amazing new modes. These cross-cultural and collapsed-time collages have inspired some of the strongest artistic innovations of recent years, creating an alternative to modernism and the more narrow post-modern paths of European and American contemporary art. Coming from the art world, I was excited to learn that Sharmila Desai was creating a similar cultural fusion in the realm of dance.

One of our recent projects at the gallery was a lecture by the French philosopher Alain Badiou, presented in collaboration with Lacanian Inc. Over the course of his talk, Badiou slowly built up a definition of art, like a sculptor constructing a sculpture. His conclusion was that art can be defined as the creation of a new form that no one has seen before. This definition is easily applied to Sharmila's work. Creating unexpected forms in her astonishing performances, she is also making art.

Jeffrey Deitch

THE SACRED DANCE OF SHARMILA DESAI

Sharmila Desai's art brings together various strains taken from the Indian tradition – among them yoga, martial arts, and the South Indian dance known as *Bharata-Natyam*. These strains can be successfully integrated because they are all devotional practices. As performed by Sharmila, dance is a ritual activity, an offering made to those higher forces which preserve the natural order and bring about its regeneration. In this reading ritual is linked to time, it provides metaphors for the gradual descent of the universe into chaos. Thus, ritual is a means of liberation, repairing damage wrought by time's passage. In the words of Ajit Mookerji, ritual is 'essentially an impulse towards reverence of the life-force and self-identification with it.' Grounded in ancient practices, it involves repeated actions and movements. Its efficacy is based on the constant repetition of prescribed gestures and actions. The Indian tradition points to numerous forms of ritual action, often performed at dawn. Daily rites often take the form of an invocation or salutation of the sun at dawn, *surya namaskar*. The most sacred of mantras, the *gayatri*, is associated with the rising sun. This yoga is often accompanied by the recitation of mantras and the practice of breathing exercises known as *pranayama*. Such techniques, taught in India over many centuries, have the effect of calming the mind through controlled breathing. First and foremost, this energy is related to the human body, hence Sharmila's focus on the body's architecture and movement as manifestations of cosmic energy.

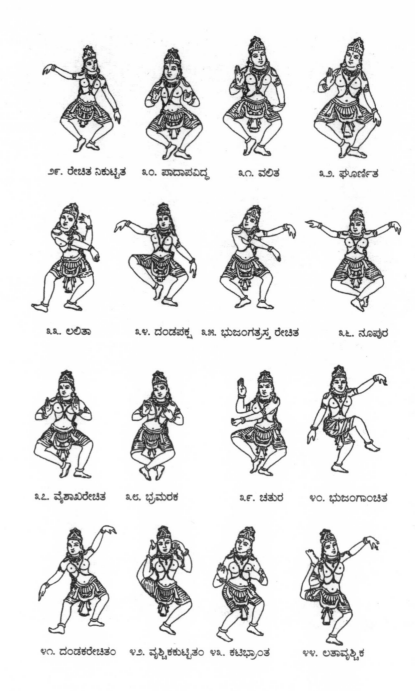

Indian dance is characterized by the idea that the creative act opens itself up to those who are allowed to witness the performer. Sharmila's dance serves as an injunction to re-live a dynamic unfolding of consciousness that has its source within as well as outside ourselves. Crucial here is the dancer's ability to create something that is capable of recreating itself within us: a strong impression that lingers and soaks up our consciousness. From this perspective we should invoke the never-ceasing dance of one of the deities in the Indian pantheon, Siva. Through his dance Siva Nataraja – the dancing Siva – recreates as well as maintains the universe in its various manifestations. He destroys by fire all earthly forms and sounds in order that creation can again be reaffirmed. This eternal dance is without a fixed point and repeats itself forever, the action never being exhausted by Siva's presence on the world-stage. All forms and bodily imprints left behind by his dance are, at best, provisional. By extension, no form created by the performer or, for that matter, perceived by the viewer, is to be accorded the character of a fixed entity. So, while each piece has a form, we acknowledge its secondary and transitory character, for it has to be integrated into the cycle of becoming – its manifestation will inevitably be followed by silence and rebirth. If this work requires the active participation of the viewer (involved in what exceeds the domain of purely auditive and retinal sensations), we reach the soteriological dimension of this art: for it to be effective, it has to penetrate to the core of our being, so that the ritual it invokes can be replicated within ourselves. Thus ritual becomes an instrument of freedom – ritual action is the result of an irrepressible dynamic.

Let us return briefly to Hindu mythology: according to the *Rg Veda*, the birth of the universe was made possible through the dismembering of a body, an original body endowed with human features called *Purusha*, the undifferentiated cosmic being. This being gave birth to the world in all its accidents and qualities from an original body and allows man, through his own actions, to reproduce and imitate this creative act. Thus, the function of ritual is to connect the two realms, microscopic and macroscopic. Sacrifice is the re-enactment of this cosmological activity. Just as this archetype of man generated the world, the individual being creates his life through his or her own ritual activity. Through discipline and symbolic sacrifice, the individual can find freedom. Through recitation, sacred dance, songs, and offerings of fruit and flowers to the temple, she sacrifices the prison of her body, the constricting dress of her Self. By turning a prescribed number of times around the altar of the temple with specific ritual gestures, the dancer integrates in her body the circles and cycles of the celestial order: she looks toward divine perfection and the place of the human being in the universe.

If energy is at the root of the manifestation of the world – as we saw, life is the result of the splitting up of a primordial being – we are invited to see life in terms of a continuous expansion and contraction of matter. This energy is replicated in the human body. The body serves as a link between the external world and the internal world: space is the common element. Contractions of breath generate an expansion of space within the body as well as in physical space. In Sanskrit there is a word for both space and sound: *Akasa*.

Movement is form that results from a particular projection or shift in space. Likewise, Sharmila's dance proceeds from a point of absolute stillness in the body and mind toward gradual expansion over time and space. As the body is subject to mutations that seem to extend the limits of its geography, the physical boundaries of the body are to be redefined. The trajectory of the body in space corresponds to an expansion in time as well: sudden shifts occur, moments of convulsion that shake the dream into which the dancer has invited us. But her dance is primarily an act of meditation: the dilation of the moment encompasses past as well as future. It reaches its plenitude when it succeeds in abolishing – or temporarily halting – the passage of time.

It is natural for us to think of time in terms of a fixed, immutable entity, along a linear pattern; whereas in India it is not unusual to conceive time in cyclical rather than linear terms. A cyclical motion is allowed to expand. Sharmila's performance plays with notions of time and space, and we realize that these are by no means fixed entities; they are elastic. Sweeping movements indicate a projection of the body in space according to a spatial and directional model. The use of postures refer to a geometry that is not only that of the human body, but finds its counterparts in the universe. Here, we find the relationship – so fundamental to Hinduism – between microcosm and macrocosm. As Karole Armitage has observed, classical dance requires speed, whereas Sharmila's choreography emphasizes the body's architecture on a geometric level. The gesture's success is related to the degree of precision that it projects; exactness then has its aesthetic quality. We do not need to know the precise significance of a particular *mudra* in order to experience the aesthetic dimension of the performance. The form of these actions traces a very specific architecture of movement.

Sharmila's choreography has the distinction of building upon the foundations of Ashtanga Vinyasa Yoga. Taught to the present day by the venerable Sri K. Pattabhi Jois, this system links breath with movement. Poses follow one another through dynamic transitions whilst the entire practice is strung together by the thread of the breath. The breath provides an evenness without which this practice would be devoid of meaning. This refers to an internal quality, but one which manifests itself externally. Following the footsteps of the legendary T. Krishnamacharya, Sri K. Pattabhi Jois has arranged the repertory of yoga *asanas* into various sequences.

A handful of postures from the various series can be identified as part of Sharmila's vocabulary. Containing countless salutations and positions, the Ashtanga system offers a gestural codification of successive movements which are always executed in the same manner, according to a spatial and directional model. The practice grows through the repetition of specific movements which, though fixed, offer unlimited potential and help shape spiritual 'becoming' by instilling the practitioner with a structure that penetrates to the core of her being. The mix of postures and the elaborate, dynamic movements linking them help redefine the architecture of the body and provide the structure of Sharmila's moves. Yet this practice is related

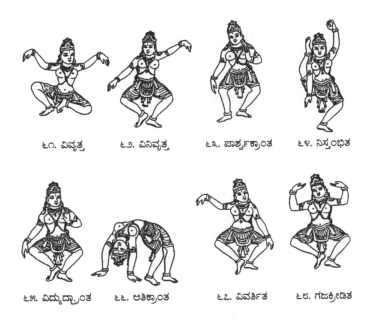

೬೧. ವಿವೃತ್ತ   ೬೨. ವಿನಿವೃತ್ತ   ೬೩. ಪಾರ್ಶ್ವಕ್ರಾಂತ   ೬೪. ನಿಸ್ತಂಭಿತ

೬೫. ವಿದ್ಯುದ್ಭ್ರಾಂತ   ೬೬. ಅತಿಕ್ರಾಂತ   ೬೭. ವಿವರ್ತಿತ   ೬೮. ಗಜಕ್ರೀಡಿತ

to dance because the sense of movement cannot be conceived without an accompanying aesthetic dimension. In addition, the quality of its realization is essential, as the work is the material repository of an inner – but by no means private – gesture or movement.

Equally familiar to Sharmila is the form of martial art known as *kalari-payattu* to which she was exposed while in Southern India. It, too, provides a blueprint for arm movements and transitions. The way to move from one stance to the next is integral to martial arts as well as to yoga. It is common to them, though technically there are differences specific to these disciplines. *Bharata-Natyam*

is an ancient dance form that originates from Tamil Nadu. It is perhaps the best known of the classical dance styles, perpetuated in modern India through schools and academies. In ancient times, dancers were linked to specific temples. It is the tradition to which Sharmila was first exposed, for her grandmother Hima Devi was a well-known *Bharata-Natyam* dancer. It provides the dancer with the root positions, both standing and sitting, as well as the essential geometry of the body's movements and lines. Special emphasis is given to the *mudras* (*mudras* are ritual positions of the hand – in Sharmila's piece *Anjali*, the *mudra* in which the two hands extended upwards are held palm to palm as in prayer form; *Anjali* means 'offering'). All these traditions are linked aesthetically. Let us also remember that *Bharata-Natyam* is considered a form of yoga that seeks union with that which is beyond all descriptions – the divine. A succession of yoga postures are to be found in the Siva dances, including the well-known *natanam adinar*. In the book of *karanas*, Siva's cosmic dance builds upon 108 yoga postures, providing yet one more link between dance and yoga. Another point of connection between these forms of corporeal expression is provided by the *dristi*, a quality of concentration, the fixing of the eyes toward particular points such as the tip of the nose, the hands or the 'third eye' (the space between the eyebrows).

Sharmila invites us to follow her into a journey of self-discovery by reinterpreting these various traditions through the ritual activity of dance. This activity is closely related to the spirit of the antique theatre. More specifically, the reenactment by humans of the actions of the gods is

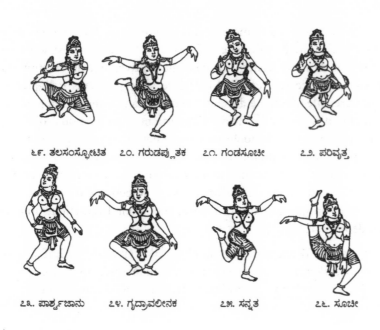

೧೯. ತಲಸಂಸ್ಫೋಟಿತ   ೨೦. ಗರುಡಪ್ಲುತಕ   ೨೧. ಗಂಡಸೂಚೀ   ೨೨. ಪರಿವೃತ್ತ

೨೩. ಪಾರ್ಶ್ವಜಾನು   ೨೪. ಗೃದ್ರಾವಲೀನಕ   ೨೫. ಸನ್ನತ   ೨೬. ಸೂಚೀ

a form of staging: the dancer strives to represent through sacrificial action the image of the cosmos of which the gods provided the model. Ritual is not only deeply tied to Sharmila's conception of art, but it offers a means of breaking away from artistic conventions. Her choreography reflects a desire to excavate the fragments of a more or less distant past, shards of memory. In this sense her work is a kind of archeology. As a form of excavation, it aims to reclaim and rewrite the deposits of this past, to salvage fragments. Her performance allows for multiple points of view and layering, as opposed to the illusion of cohesive unity, or a retreat into a lost tradition. This lost terrain can only

be recreated through an act of imagination. India's traditions are not merely being replayed or evoked, but reinvented as the dancer traces her journey through time and space: time suspended, space conquered. It is through this act of imagination that she attains aesthetic and formal freedom.

For *Anjali*, Sharmila devised a choreography in three movements: invocation, rapture, surrender; the corresponding colors on the set were gold amber, fuchsia and blue, with a musical score that fused a recorded soundtrack by Cheb i Sabah with live improvisation by two South Indian percussionists. In *Arati*, a piece dedicated to the art of Yves Klein, Sharmila devised a sequence that took its inspiration from the sun salutations of Ashtanga Vinyasa Yoga (which are not unlike the salutations that Yves Klein learned as a devoted Judoka) and the sun invocation of *kalari payattu*. For Klein, too, art was conceived as a ritual which has its root in ancient sacrificial cults that are to be renewed daily in order for us to find appeasement. Such art has an aim that is not only aesthetic, but also therapeutic. Through imagination and skill, the rhythms of daily life are recreated, offering an eloquent image of the endless cycle of becoming. There is joy in this activity. With Sharmila's dance, the reconfiguration of the body's language into seemingly effortless but vertiginous directions provides a sense of exhilaration, so little aware as we are to the body's possibilities, while we realize that this magical unfolding is steeped in ancient knowledge.

Olivier Berggruen

BIOGRAPHY

Sharmila Desai comes from a family of dancers, most notably her great aunt Menaka and her grandmother Hima Devi, who were legendary exponents of dance. Similar to her predecessors in pushing traditional forms of movement and art, Desai has intermingled martial art, yoga and Indian dance to explore ancient ideas in the realm of the contemporary. Notable recent performances include the Venice Biennale, Deitch Projects, ICA London and the opening for the Yves Klein Retrospective at the Schirn Kunsthalle Frankfurt.

PLATE LIST

COVER – Photo by Briana Blasko, costume by VPL, signature by Sanyucta Desai **PLATE I** – The home of Sharmila's father Goa, India circa 1940 **PLATE II** – Shahzia Sikander Bound, 2001 Color photogravure with soft ground etching and spit bite and water bite aquatints 18 1/4 x 14 1/2 inches, edition 25 Published by Crown Point Press **PLATE III** – Sharmila's great aunt Menaka and dancer circa 1930 **PLATE IV** – Left page: Menaka with dancers circa 1930 Right page: Menaka at Rabindranath Tagore's Shantiniketan in Calcutta circa 1930; Photograph of Sharmila by Suran Goonatilake © **PLATE V** – Left page: Photo of Sharmila by Suran Goonatilake © Right page: Menaka circa 1930 **PLATE VI** – Menaka circa 1930 **PLATE VII** – Photo of Sharmila by Suran Goonatilake © **PLATE VIII** – Menaka circa 1930 **PLATE IX** – Photo of Sharmila by Suran Goonatilake © **PLATE X** – Photo of Sharmila by Suran Goonatilake © **PLATE XI** – Photo of Sharmila by Suran Goonatilake © **PLATE XII** – Ganges River at Gangotri taken by Sharmila Desai during her trek to Gomukh 2002 **PLATE XIII** – Live performance photos of Sharmila taken at the Schirn Kunsthalle Museum, Frankfurt, Germany: Premiere of 'ARATI' for the opening of the Yves Klein Retrospective September 17, 2004 Curated by Olivier Berggruen and Max Hollein **PLATE XIV** – Live performance photos of Sharmila by Maciej Rusinek **PLATE XV** – Somnathpur, India 2002 **PLATE XVI** – 'Out of blue' live performance at the Tang Museum in collaboration with Shahzia Sikkander January 30, 2004 Curated by Ian Berry **PLATE XVII** – Photo of Sharmila by Suran Goonatilake © **PLATE XVIII** – Aarti in Haridwar, India 2002 by SD **PLATE XIX** – Photo of Sharmila by Suran Goonatilake © **PLATE XX** – Tiruvanamalai, India 2002 by SD **PLATE XXI** – Live performance at the Aldrich Museum in collaboration with Shahzia Sikkander September 19, 2004 Curated by Jessica Hough **PLATE XXII** – Live performance at the Aldrich Museum in collaboration with Shahzia Sikkander September 19, 2004 Curated by Jessica Hough **PLATE XXIII** – Live performance at the Aldrich Museum in collaboration with Shahzia Sikkander September 19, 2004 Curated by Jessica Hough **PLATE XXIV** – Photo by Vanina Sorrenti for I-D Magazine 25th anniversary, clothes by VPL **PLATE XXV** – Photo by Vanina Sorrenti for I-D Magazine 25th anniversary **PLATE XXVI** – Photo by Briana Blasko, costume by VPL Riverside Park 2005 **PLATE XXVII** – Tiruvanamalai, India 2002 by SD **PLATE XXVIII** – Live performance at ICA, London, U.K. 1999 **PLATE XXIX** – Video projection during live performance by Mo-ling Chui, Deitch Projects 2003 **PLATE XXX** – Video stills by Shankar Desai, Deitch Projects 2003 **PLATE XXXI** – Live performance for Akanksha benefit - proceeds to program working with street children programs in Bombay Organized by Anita Trehan and Sarah Roberts **PLATE XXXII** – Live performance for Akanksha benefit - proceeds to program working with street children programs in Bombay Organized by Anita Trehan and Sarah Roberts **PLATE XXXIII** – Live performance for the Tibetan Peace Garden Benefit Wiltshire, U.K. **PLATE XXXIV** – Live Performance at Schirn Kunsthalle Museum Frankfurt, Germany. Mridangam by Vidwan Bangalore R. N. Prakash, Ghatam & Moorsing by Pirashanna Thevaraja, projections by Mo-ling Chui set design by Sanyucta Desai **PLATE XXXV** – Live performance at Schirn Kunsthalle Museum Frankfurt, Germany **PLATE XXXVI** – Live performance at Deitch Projects light design by Paul Breen **PLATE XXXVII** – The home of Sharmila's paternal grandmother Goa, India circa 1950 **PLATE XXXVIII** – Photo of Sharmila by Suran Goonatilake © **PLATE XXXIX** – Temple at Bal Ganga, Mumbai, India 2002 **PLATE XL** – Photo by Vanina Sorrenti **PLATE XLI** – Audubon Park New Orleans, Louisiana 2005 **PLATE XLII** – Photo by Vanina Sorrenti **PLATE XLIII** – Goa, India circa 1950 **PLATE XLIV** – Photo by Brooke Slezak 2003 **PLATE XLV** – The home of Sharmila's father Goa, India circa 1950 **PLATE XLVI** – Shahzia Sikander Elusive Realities #1, 2000 Acrylic on canvas 120 x 80 inches Image courtesy of Sikkema Jenkins & Co.; Photo by Jaishri Abichandani **PLATE XLVII** – Select drawings from the 108 Shiva Karanas

Printed in Italy by Grafiche Antiga - Cornuda, Treviso